Living with the Other Side

Answers to Life are Within You

Noel Harding

First published by Busybird Publishing 2022

Copyright © 2022 Noel Harding

ISBN
978-1-922691-38-5 (paperback)
978-1-922691-39-2 (ebook)

This work is copyright. Apart from any use permitted under the *Copyright Act 1968*, no part of this publication may be reproduced, stored in a retrieval system or transmitted in any form or by any means, electronic, mechanical, photocopying, recording or otherwise, without the prior written permission of Noel Harding.

Cover Image: Shane Miller (non contactable)

Cover design: Busybird Publishing

Layout and typesetting: Busybird Publishing

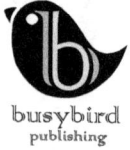

Busybird Publishing
2/118 Para Road
Montmorency, Victoria
Australia 3094
www.busybird.com.au

Dedicated to my family.

Other books by Noel Harding:

Fine Line

Contents

Note From the Author 1

Chapter 1
The Other Side of Life 5

Chapter 2
Our Hidden Self 9

Chapter 3
Ego. The 'I, Me and My' -
Our Best Friend and Worst Enemy 19

Chapter 4
The Real Me Within 29

Chapter 5
Dreams -
Nightmares, Soul, Feelings, Precognition or All 43

Chapter 6
My Personal Myths -
What is Your Personal Myth? 59

Chapter 7
The Blues 65

Chapter 8
Negative Energies, Positive Energies and Feelings 83

Chapter 9
The Troll Under the Bridge 97

Chapter 10
The Big Movers 105

Chapter 11
Confrontation with the Unconscious (Universe)   109

Chapter 12
In The Arms of The Universe   115

Acknowledgements   125
References   127

Note From the Author

The original idea for this book is simply to pass on to my 'family' information and techniques I have spent my whole adult life seeking and putting into action.

If a simple working-class boy, with assistance from mentors and education, can learn to look at and begin to understand the power of the unconscious, then anybody can.

Some may ask with what authority I can write on such a subject. My answer is simply, apart from the formal and spiritual studies I have done in these areas, my main teacher has been life. I have endeavoured to live and put into action, even in my business ventures, all I speak about. Most of the time my intellect and ego hampered my relationship with higher aspects of myself. My ego, however, did provide contrast, a necessary driver for inner growth. When all reasoning failed and my foxy ego had control, only through dreams and active meditation have I been able to directly find what propels and inspires me, positively and negatively.

I met my life teacher when I was twenty-three. That's when the 'trouble' started. He believed that all religions have a common denominator of good and that the individualisation of men and women is of the utmost importance. The journey into knowing oneself, on one hand, is a serious, disciplined, relentless search. On the other hand, it is a natural human endeavour where humour plays a very necessary part.

Some, including myself, may point the finger and say, 'Noel Harding, he is far from perfect'. And I would reply, 'Isn't that the point? Life is all about growing. I want to grow, but growing sometimes involves painful mistakes.'

There is a beauty and wisdom deep within all of us that we have a right to experience. Each of us is uniquely different, originating from different cultures, life experiences, and family ancestral roots. Once these basic facts are accepted, judging of oneself and others begins to diminish.

On one hand the subject matter ventures where angels fear to tread, but at the same time, it is down to earth, practical and common sense. The only other prerequisites required to really want to know yourself are a little guts, the need to change, and the ability to question conventional thinking.

Through our lives we care, we pain, we love, we grow. The true and real we seek; the best is always known.

Madness of love's mirrored perfection blinds as childhood experiences, fears and symbols all merge together on the winding way to the future.

Beyond all, ever-present love, understanding love, moves through the mist as woman and man, hand by hand, are invited to climb the mountain of the self.

NH

An enlightened first century Roman, trying to navigate the complexities of that time said, 'I have avoided shame, but I deserve no praise.'

Chapter
1

The Other Side of Life

How often have we reached and grasped at answers to life, or for that matter, for answers to our daily problems, only to find our reasoning ability, our intellect, our conscious ego, the 'I, me and my' part of us, leading us firmly along paths which leave us more frustrated and confused than before. Maybe the answers lie elsewhere.

To some people the unconscious part of the mind is the darker side of the moon, even demonic. To others it can be an unlimited source of balance, beauty and creativity, even of spirituality. For most of us, until we learn to understand, tap into, utilise and learn to live with this massive storehouse of information and energy, we just edge around this beautiful, bottomless, volcanic-like lake of magic, occasionally dipping in our big toe or falling out of control into its mysterious all-consuming waters.

What is this unconscious made of? Is there really something there or is it all just a myth, a fairy story or a figment of our imagination? Is the unconscious a personal thing, a deep record of everything that has happened to us, something we share with others, or a complex combination of the two? If we do accept an unconscious may exist, is it neutral, does it embody love and compassion, is it static or is it continually changing? Does this secret area of our minds have the ability to right itself and hold balance? Is our unconscious the sum total of all we have put into it as individuals in our lives? Does it contain content from before we were born, from our, and other generations? Does our unconscious require continual input or dogma?

Is the unconscious blank and neutral, a mere record of memory, just an accumulation of positive and negative past events? Is it influenced by a higher power or higher area of our minds?

If we look at all cultures and races throughout the world it is obvious that humans have a need to practice communicating with this mysterious side of their minds. It would seem that every race, community, and individual, in one way or another, seeks the excitement, comfort, healing, inspiration, and to some, the destruction that can be accessed from this deeper side of our existence. We will look together at how this eternal storehouse within, continually motivates us, continually mystifies, frustrates, serves and inspires us both at the individual communal levels, worldwide and possibly beyond.

We have all had the experience of being transported to another place. It may be after we visit the movies, listen to music, when we dream, fall in love, go to church, or experience hypnosis. It may be when we are involved in the birth of a child or the death of someone close, when we take a short cut with drugs, alcohol or just daydream. How and why can we be moved to another place? Why is it so different, so scary, so magical? One thing that can't be denied is, like an iceberg floating in the ocean, the human mind has a lot going on below the surface.

In a practical way this book incorporates age-old techniques and brings them into the present, harnesses and puts to work the insights and energies from those hidden magic parts of ourselves. As a result, the world as we have been experiencing it, can change forever. We can go back, look at the past, and alter its effects on us. We can also set new goals and outcomes for the future. Time can be condensed and expanded.

Carl Jung, a renowned Swiss investigator of the unconscious, a one-time close friend of Sigmund Freud, believed that the only way to know the self and develop into a whole individual human being is to understand the unconscious at all its levels. But even he admitted, 'There is only so far we can go, the unconscious goes on to infinity.' (Jung, 1963).

Know yourself. With some simple insights and procedures, you can be in control of your own destiny and be your own doctor of the psyche. Jung maintained that, 'The individual who wishes to have an answer to the complexities of life, as it is posed today, needs first and foremost, of self-knowledge, that is, the utmost acknowledgement of his own wholeness. He or she should know relentlessly how much good they can do, and what crimes they are capable of, and must beware of regarding one as real and the other as illusion. Both are elements within his or her nature, and both are bound to come to light within, should it be wished.'

A simple roadmap does exist. It's my aim to demonstrate, using life experiences of you, myself and others, to show how any person can take preventative control over their own destiny without the ongoing support of organised groups or sometimes, 'unnecessary' psychological counselling.

There are some shortcuts, but mostly it takes guts, relaxation, motivation and application. The past, present and the future go hand in hand. We know how the past influences the future. The past as we see it, can be understood, accepted and changed. Remember the past is as far away as the last sentence you have just read, and the future, the next sentence you may read.

Chapter 2

Our Hidden Self

If we acknowledge there is a vast storehouse of information, instincts and feelings available to us constantly, logic would suggest that all our life experiences and perceptions cannot be in the forefront of our minds every minute of the day. It would seem humans have developed a filtering or filing system which protects our day-to-day mind from being overrun by a myriad of unrelenting, seemingly unnecessary information. Should we stir all this up? Haven't we got enough to contend with? Is there any point in delving? What is to be gained? Can it be dangerous?

If we look for organic proof that access to the unconscious is ok, dreams are our evidence of a natural, everyday, direct communication we all have with our unconscious.

It's important to understand how you can use your unconscious, but it's also crucial that you are aware how others can use your deeper side to waylay or take advantage of you.

Carl Jung talks about archetypes. He has defined them as powerful, unconscious groups of energies which have common themes and exist right across the board in the psyche of all humans individually. Throughout his practicing and private life, he has observed, grouped and labelled these powerful energies, maintaining they are constantly directing and influencing us moment by moment, most times without us being aware. Politicians, artists, film makers, advertisers, religious leaders, writers, editors, promoters and the military use these unconscious motivators, either purposely or inadvertently to achieve their positive or negative ends. One of Carl Jung's archetypes, the symbol of the child, constantly reassures and motivates some of us with its promise of new life or new beginning. The Christ child has symbolised hope and love to the western world for the last two thousand years.

It is common for young soldiers to be trained, sent to war feeling heroic and invincible, and then spend the rest of their adult lives, if they survive, wondering where all that youthful bravado came from. It is known that men, from age seventeen to their early twenties, are physically strong and mentally mouldable. Jung would term this unconscious predisposition, the hero archetype. It is potentially present in a large percentage of men and women.

One of the most troubling and dangerous situations has always been where intelligent leaders, even democratically elected, convinced that they have got it right, use powerful unconscious energies and symbols to motivate masses of people. Throughout history we have seen these intelligent, persuasive people constantly get it wrong, instigating conflicts where many suffer. This still continues to this very hour.

Varying differences leading to prejudices and misunderstanding can exist between cultures and whole countries. A leader can give in to destructive negativity within an individual, group or a whole population and use it to manipulate. A strong leader, however, will always seek new and positive directions even if it goes against popular belief.

At the individual level, each and every one of us can identify basic human tendencies, understand if we are being influenced positively or negatively, and then make a decision whether or not we want to continue accepting the same old same old. The power of some of these influences should not be underestimated. Think about how groups and individuals around you use these powerful energies to manipulate you, your family and others to further their own wealth or power base. In the end, manipulators of man and womankind must understand, there is an old saying, 'You can fool some people some of the time, but you can't fool all of the people all of the time.'

Ways We are Manipulated

- Fear: What individuals, groups or organisations use fear to motivate us?

- Greed: Who appeals to the greedy aspect of us?

- Sex: Are you aware when you are being motivated by sex?

- Food: Which companies are guilty of marketing unnecessarily expensive or unhealthy foods?

- Peace: Do we fall for false promises of peace and tranquillity?

- Power: What makes you feel powerful and which organisations market power?

- Beauty: The association between you and physical beauty – who promotes this?

- Hero worship: Who makes you feel heroic and why?

- Love and compassion: Are there organisations that pray on your loving and compassionate side and profit from this?

Why should others have the ability to understand and motivate us using our unconscious hidden positive or negative energies? Why should others be in control? The way to stop your deeper side from being misused by others and yourself is to know your inner self through and through.

There appears to be many levels within the unconscious. Our dreams can show us this clearly. We all know some dreams tend to deal with day-to-day stuff, others can come from deeper levels and rock us at our very foundations. Simple dreams that reflect day to day conflicts, fears and wish fulfilments, we may think about and take note and disregard as we shower. But there are other dreams that stay with us for hours or days, dreams that repeat over and over, dreams that seem to tell us the future, and there are a few dreams which we never forget. We then have nightmares. Even those are explainable unless they have dietary or chemical influence.

Happiness, sorrow, conflicts and our instincts seem to sit in the background, in our subconscious, and either pop forward without any warning or are triggered by some small thought, or life trigger. How often have you thought that it was just a dream and laid the experience to one side? It is very likely, however, you have tapped into and experienced bubble-ups from one of these elusive layers of your subconscious self, and not necessarily by chance.

Throughout our lives, when things are going well and there are no dramas or extremes, everything appears to sit tightly and securely in its place. It is only when trauma or excitement stirs us emotionally that we find a great deal more lies just below the surface. These underlying energies or manifestations, under certain circumstances, can be identified by what seems a premonition, a predictive (precognitive) dream or seeming coincidence. A person familiar with reading the underlying areas of the mind can be referred to as psychic. Each of us have our intuitive moments, moments when we lift above all the prattle and can see things very clearly. All of us have our own small psychic moments and stories to tell.

When troubles in life come along, as they do, some of us turn to so-called psychics for answers. Even royalty and world leaders, both for positive and negative reasons, have in the past, and still do, turn to clairvoyants.

During the Second World War, Churchill consulted clairvoyants and used their information (Willis). In moments of desperation, how many times have others turned to you for help, a listening ear, and another point of view which is separate from their temporary confusion? When we choose a person to confide in it's usually somebody, at that point in time, who can see past our 'I, me and myself' and help us to contact that steadiness within, which, in retrospect, usually seems to have been there all the time. Wouldn't it be great to be able to contact this incorruptible part of ourselves without relying on others with their varying ideas and their unique life perceptions to steady us? It's possible. Let's move outside our square and investigate if these levels of unconsciousness exist. How to identify these bubble-ups from the layers of our unconscious, befriend them, not fear them, and put them to work in a positive and constructive way. This can be tricky, but is definitely achievable.

The whole point is we don't have to look too far. The energies are right here with us every day. Should the subconscious scare us? No, because our subconscious is our very own, to do with as we wish. Just like the part of us that tells our body how to breathe, digest food, make internal body repairs, and walk without thinking about it, this stream of energy, positive and sometimes negative, is constantly working in the background. For example, just as we can involuntarily influence, with worry, stress and excitement, the medulla of the brain that controls our heart rate. We can learn to modify parts of these hidden areas to change and protect us.

Psychologists, religious leaders, psychics, advertisers and leaders of primitive races all seem to acknowledge that a very powerful area of the mind lies just below our day-to-day conscious state. Why does the ordinary man and woman separate themselves from this other side? Why do we leave it to the so-called experts? After all, our unconscious is an intrinsic part of our individual being, why should others try to delve into, control and influence it?

Why do we shy away from the deeper part of our being? 'It's scary, leave it to the experts' we may say. 'I'm not qualified. I don't have the skills or the training. It's dangerous to delve' the professionals may say. There are no rules. Each and every one of us has the right to explore that deeper part of our nature which influences us every moment of the day and night, even whilst we sleep.

Some who have knowledge of the workings of the unconscious refuse to empower the individual to affect his or her own internal growth. Instead, individuals are made reliant and encouraged to allow decisions to be made for them. In the external world this has constant ramifications in the areas of the environment, personal health, our relationship with other cultures, education, and the relationship between men and women.

Is it possible to free up and take control of our own individual lives and destinies? The answer is yes. Where do we start? What is the closest identifiable source of unconscious information about ourselves which is personally and readily available?

Dreams and meditation are our direct link with our unconscious. Each time we sleep a small window or door opens into another world. Those of us who can remember our dreams, most times take this experience for granted until we stop and think about it. You may say 'I don't dream'. But it has been scientifically proven we all dream even if we don't remember. There may be reasons our dreams are blocked, or it could just be a case of some focusing or application of a little technique, such as placing a pad and pen beside our bed with the intention to record our dreams.

We have all heard of the term meditation and for most of us that's where it starts and finishes. It sounds like a complex procedure reserved for those who are 'advanced souls' or 'the super sensitive'. Again, this is not the case. We all can drop into a state of meditation, and most of us do on a daily basis. Day dreaming or 'being off with the fairies' is a form of hypnosis or meditation which all of us can switch in and out of very quickly. Children do it all the time. Simple techniques for going into hypnosis, deep relaxation, meditation or prayer to achieve relaxation, communicate with our higher-self, change parts of our unwanted behaviours or improve our self-image will also be covered in detail later.

Emotions and feelings visit us on a daily basis both in dreams and in our awake state. Some are negative and others positive, or that is the way it seems. We may be tempted to think that this only happens to me, but the more we talk to people about feelings and emotions, the more we realise there is a great deal more going on in our minds than is always obvious. Later, we will talk about understanding and accepting negative feelings and how to view and convert them for positive use.

Signalling out, identifying and dealing with unconscious 'bubble ups' which can take the form of free-floating anxieties, fantasies, fears, desires and archetypal* influences, is another way of using subconscious messages to improve your understanding about yourself and how you interact with others.

It is not difficult to recognise negative and positive energies within us, separate them out and see them for what they are. Putting yourself in control by removing unnecessary fear is not as difficult as some would make out.

In later chapters we will also look at many simple ways to connect with, live with, and work with the unconscious, that magical untapped other side of ourselves.

*Jungian term for groups of energies which he maintains are common human group psychic energies existing, across cultures, in the unconscious. (Jung, 1963)

Chapter
3

Ego. The 'I, Me and My'
Our Best Friend and Worst Enemy

In the first years of our lives, for our protection and development, the 'I, me and my' part of ourselves, our ego, is developed and reinforced by our family and/or significant others. 'You are a good girl', 'What a smart boy you are', 'Don't you look beautiful', 'Aren't you strong'. These are messages of encouragement that emanate from that special, constructive, caring side of ourselves, instinctively nurturing and wanting the best for an offspring.

From our early years, the 'I' aspect of ourselves, the ego, is formed, developed and entrenched. Once the concept of the self, our 'I, me or my' is established, we are then encouraged to change, consider others, and the social structure in which we live, and cohesively co-exist within the world of opposites and contradictions.

The ego or the 'I' part of us tries to make sense of the world and guide us. We do the best we can, but it is difficult for most of us to see things objectively from a distance. Our upbringing, culture, and even education can override our true self and continue to reinforce the entrenchment of the 'I, me and my'. It would seem we all have great difficulty in breaking free from the infantile self-centred parts of ourselves. We may think our ego protects us from a world that is not always kind, and in the past, it may feel that it probably has. But it can also draw us into conflict, interfere with our ability to see from the point of view of others, and stop us from standing back and seeing the bigger picture.

Our ego has been a good friend, sometimes our only friend. It has been a source of information, reassurance, pleasure and security. Is it possible to find answers from another place, a place which is unaffected by selfishness and complex, blinkered half-truths? How much 'I, me and my' input do we really need in our lives? Is it an alternative to be humble, and, if so, how vulnerable does this make us? Does it mean we put everybody else's needs before our own? Should we eliminate material things and the enjoyments modern living and technology brings? No, this is not what uncovering the higher aspects of ourselves is about.

Is there a relationship between our 'I, me and my' parts of ourselves, and our self-esteem? They can both be very different. An individual with a high developing self-esteem usually has the ability to put him or herself in the shoes of the other person. As a result of working with their inner self, an individual can develop an ever-increasing calming, intuitive and balanced outlook. When the foxy ego is influencing our communication and our actions, we all know what can happen. The way we view things is limited by our perceptions. We judge, we don't listen, our empathy diminishes and invariably we can rush in where angels fear to tread.

You may wonder how to begin to understand the unconscious aspects of my ego? How will this affect those around me? Deep down everybody will respect your endeavours, however, once you set your course it is an individual process which may confuse some around you.

My Declaration of Self-esteem
(Unknown author)

I am me.

In the entire world, there is no one else exactly like me. There are people who have some parts like me, but no one adds up exactly as I do. Therefore, everything that comes out of me is authentically mine because I alone choose it.

I own everything about me – my body, including everything it does; my mind, including all its thoughts and ideas; my eyes, including all the images they behold; my feelings whatever they may be – anger, joy, frustration, love disappointment, excitement; my mouth and all the words that come out of it, polite, sweet or rough, correct or incorrect; my voice, loud or soft; and all my actions, whether they be to others or to myself.

I own my fantasies, my dreams, my hopes, my fears.

I own all my triumphs and successes, all my failures and mistakes.

Because I own all of me, I can become intimately acquainted with me. By doing so, I can love me and be friendly with me in all my parts. I can then make it possible for all of me to work in its best interests.

I know there are aspects about myself that puzzle me, and other aspects I do not know. But as long as I am friendly and loving to myself, I can courageously and hopefully look for solutions to the puzzles and for ways to find out more about me.

However I look and sound, whatever I say and do, and whatever I think and feel at a given moment in time, is me. This is authentic and represents where I am at that moment in time.

When I review later how I looked and sounded, what I said and did, and how I thought and felt, some parts may turn out to be unfitting. I can discard that which is unfitting, and keep that which proved fitting, and invent something new for that which I discarded.

> *I can see, hear, feel, think, say and do. I have tools to survive, to be close to others, to be productive, and to make sense and order out of the world of people and things outside of me.*
>
> *I own me, and therefore I can engineer me.*
>
> *I am me and I am okay.*

If we are going to move away from a self-centred life to that of a broader outlook, where do we start, what are our reference points? Do we learn about understanding the ego from those who try to crush it with dogma? Can we be enlightened by idealists who give or fight until they are weary or disillusioned? Can we glean any truth from those who retreat to caves or monasteries cutting themselves off from the real world? Can those who never enter into ongoing relationships, such as monks and priests, ever understand the day-to-day complex feelings and situations that can arise? Sometimes it may be possible.

The answers are within each of us. We all make decisions daily which determine the direction we will go for the next hour, the next day, the next year, sometimes for a lifetime. It is very easy to say, 'why should I take the hard option? Nobody else does.' We might say, 'that's the way things are – I can't change the world.'

The ego, which should not be confused with our deeper self, is very cunning. When everything is going the way that our inner cunning ego wants, there is no resistance. Like the Gingerbread man, a mythical children's story character, part of us can be duped by our selfish needs and perceptions until exhausted and our health is affected.

Why did the Gingerbread man want to go to the other side of the river? Why did he climb onto a fox's back? Why was he so weak and reliant in the first place? Why did he hand his life and destiny over to a fox? For whatever reason he needed to seek greener pastures, on the other side of the river and fell victim to the charisma of the fox who offered to carry him there. The fox could represent the human ego seducing our little character, made from ginger and shortbread, who is honest, kind but vulnerable, following his dream. The fox goes into deeper and deeper water forcing the Gingerbread man, who cannot get wet, onto his shoulder closer and closer to the fox's mouth.

Our egos do slowly seduce our higher attributes causing pain, illness and sometimes our premature demise. The egos of the world's great manipulators can cause massive suffering, even to this very day. Because he was the Gingerbread man, fragile and prone to taking shortcuts he was vulnerable. Maybe the story ends well, but, what we have to consider is the time factor. How much time do we spend with the pendulum swinging between selfish needs and our higher faculties?

What effect does this have on our health, the people around us and the future of the planet?

Enough of the questions and theory. In the next chapter we will look at how to go into a relaxed state – a state of hypnosis or meditation – in order to alter aspects of behaviour. For now, here is a short exercise which helps to identify and separate out the influences of the ego. Expectations or needs are difficult to change immediately, but just to challenge a previous mind set may be a good start. How would you handle the following life situations?

1. You are on a cruise with twenty-five other people. The sailboat sinks, the waters are below freezing and the lifeboat definitely only has room for fifteen. Bringing another aboard would risk the lives of everybody in the boat. You are in the life boat and five others are in the water holding onto the side. What would you do? One of those in the water could be a family member.

2. You have an excellent career. One of your fellow workmates is wrongfully having their self-esteem intensely abused by your employer. To take sides or to challenge your boss could result in you losing your job. What would you do?

3. You are at a restaurant. Your favourite cake is served, one piece is larger, but

it is not obvious. Without any health considerations, which piece would you choose and why?

4. You are walking down the street and you come across somebody brutally kicking another person unconscious. How would you handle the situation?

When you consider your responses, from what part of your mind are you attempting to find an answer? Was your solution instantaneous or did you have to labour over it? Did the answers have a common theme of self-preservation, one of self-sacrifice, indifference, or a combination of all? Whatever, it's the mind's process that we can note. Some of the above situations are extreme, but every day we make hundreds of decisions that determine what happens that day, that week and sometimes decisions that will affect us for a lifetime. How fast we drive, how many alcoholic drinks, undermining a person's self-esteem with regrettable words, actions and inactions. Where do wrong decisions emanate from? How often have we all wished we could take back something we said, or could erase a past action?

Have you ever made the comments or thought, 'I am not perfect' and 'I've done the best I can'? These are very human responses to life situations, but it is interesting to think about the origins of such thoughts and comments. Let's look at the phrase, 'I am not perfect,' when it originates from the 'I, me and my' part of ourselves. Our cunning ego, trying to stay in control, can sometimes subtly convince us to take a short-cut, to compromise, leading to those disappointing consequences we are all too familiar with. The same thought or comment emanating from our higher-self or wise mind can put a totally different slant on, 'I'm not perfect.' It could mean, 'I haven't achieved what I wanted, but I tried and will do better next time,' or 'I give myself permission to make mistakes.'

How can communication with our unconscious-self have anything to do with our decision making? If we agree that our decisions are sometimes negatively influenced from deeper areas of our mind, we can't quite put our finger on it, then maybe we can use this same area of our mind to find answers that lead to a less stressful and more peaceful, productive, confident approach to life.

The following chapter specifically sets out simple procedures and exercises, not usually publicised, which will equip any individual, motivated to change, to communicate with his or her innate, unconscious inner energies.

A subsequent chapter discusses converting negative energies, feelings and seeming positive feelings to positive.

Chapter 4

The Real Me Within

This chapter simply and specifically demonstrates how to use suggestions and affirmations, in conjunction with deep relaxation exercises, to achieve baby steps on the way to improving self-esteem and behaviours.

Beyond all, your self-esteem needs to be intact, you have to love and respect yourself if you want to be respected, get along with others and not be manipulated. It is not the aim of this chapter to deal with phobias (irrational fears) or everyday psychological problems, although they can be dealt with using hypnosis and deep relaxation therapy with the help of a therapist. As inner strength and love for oneself develops, unwanted habits tend to fall away and a natural inclination to tackle psychological things are less daunting and easier than ever before.

Self-esteem deficiencies can manifest in many different ways. Low self-esteem is where an individual is convinced they have no self-worth or very little, sometimes with reason, sometimes perceived. Then there's the Gatsby/Walter Mitty type, those living in a dream world of imagined or actual achievements believing the material life, or world of daydreams, makes the individual. The intellectual who feels everything can be solved by reasoning, education and brain power. And there are those of us who repress some life guilts, perceived physical deficiencies or actual traumas, which progressively erodes feelings of self-worth, but paradoxically can inspire great personal endeavours. There are accomplished individuals who have a perceived or imagined low self-image, no achievement or reassurance is enough placing immense pressure on themselves and others around them. We may all have experienced variations on these feelings, but don't we all still, deep down, strive for balance?

Influences emanating from ancestors or previous generations can be magical gifts or the most unwanted negative energies. Understanding these passed-on influences and developing an objective, protective empathy for the negatives, or seeming negatives, allows the magic aspects of our inherited ancestral achievements to complement our journey and subsequently what we pass onto our children.

The types of basic exercises we will be using are adopted in similar form, worldwide, by athletes, psychologists, business individuals, hypnotherapists and spiritual aspirants. Carried out consistently and with honest, genuine intent, the exercises will bring deep change within. However, as with any preventative practices, trust, perseverance and the ability to hang in there when nothing appears to be happening, is essential. Further use of simple exercises to eliminate unwanted negative behaviours will also be covered in a later chapter.

Some things we should be aware of at the outset: It is the aim of these exercises to strike a balance within and empower you, the individual, and to make you un-reliant on anything or anybody else. Using your personal 'spiritual' or higher intuition during the course of these exercises will prove more successful than an approach from your ego side – your 'I, me and my'. Simply, this means putting all self-centred feelings, habits and notions, temporarily, in a box and putting them to one side. Remember your personal symbols and day-dreams, which will be used in the course of the exercises, cannot be of a general nature: each of us is original and different. Our life symbols are uniquely, individually our own. A brief, simple reason for this is that some would consider a park or the sea general symbols of peace and tranquillity and could be used in relaxation sessions or visualisations. How wrong could this be if you had been raped in a park or nearly drowned in the ocean?

From the day we are born and prior to that through ancestral, communal experiences, through DNA, folklore, nursery rhymes, cave paintings, stories, religion and books, our unique personal traits and symbols are developed and stored deep within each of us. These combined with our life-generated symbols and various modellings from family and mentors may come into play and work in parallel.

It is best to do the following exercises as prevention rather than an immediate cure, using your choice of day-dreams and personal symbols. Deep relaxation is the key and there is no place for negative feelings or thoughts during any of the exercises. You will find, like an uninvited person to a party, the negative thoughts will stay away. When you are depressed or if you are mentally challenged is not the time to attempt to alter deeper aspects of yourself. Seek qualified assistance.

Western medicine has made incredible gains in the curative side of medicine. We have become accustomed to immediate cures and results. With adjustments to self-esteem and behaviour modification, the progress of change may be imperceptible, even though it is taking place. Negative behaviours, most times, form over a long period of our life and we are strongly influenced by those who have come before us. So be persistent, patient and strong.

Carry out the exercises when you are feeling positive and happy. Definitely not if you are depressed. It is not necessary for you to be completely convinced the affirmations and suggestions you will be using are a reality for you at present, they are your positive day-dreams coming from the real you, nourished with additional exercises, like seeds once planted, they will grow. Remember the good stuff has always been there and it wants to flourish. How do we know this? Most humans want the best for their offspring, in spite of their own failings. We see this demonstrated every day. The best feelings are also relative to your inner child.

In a later chapter we will look at transmuting negative feelings and energies to positive.

The exercises should be approached as if your visualisation/day-dreams/aspirations have actually been accomplished, e.g. A sample suggestion, *'I am a confident individual with a high self-esteem.'* Not, *'I want to be a confident individual* … The first is a strong suggestion, the second could imply defeat. The use of the word 'try' also implies defeat and should always be avoided. Finally, when we give ourselves a suggestion or create a visualisation, our brains, when in a deep relaxation state, absorb the positive message much more potently than if we just think about it at the day-to-day conscious level. The relaxed state allows the messages to penetrate into our subconscious and slowly, but surely, become embedded in new behaviour.

Here are a cross section of example affirmations and visualisations. They may be similar to your symbols and daydreams. However, the very essence and accuracy of the exercises relies on you using your own personal symbols and expressions of your needs and requirements – your own personal myth content – your inner motivating forces.

- I am a healthy, strong individual with a high self-esteem.

- I am a relaxed, empathic person, trustworthy and a good listener.

- I am a unique, strong and giving, balanced individual.

- I am a sincere, accepting, happy individual.

- I am a healthy, fearless individual with a positive self-image.

- I am a balanced person with strength and empathy for myself and others.

- I am vibrant, happy and I love myself.

The techniques we will be using to modify unwanted behaviours and embellish existing positives can be used anywhere. For example, on an aeroplane, on a bus, in a crowd, even in a panic situation, but initially find a quiet place.

Let's go: There are many ways you can enter a deep state of relaxation; this is one. Initially, sit in a relaxed position, back straight, head upright, two feet on the floor. Put either arm out at a little above 45 degrees and let it go limp at the wrist. Close your eyes, roll them up a little under your eyelids and concentrate on feeling the weight of your arm. Your arm will become heavier and heavier. Tell yourself to relax your legs, relax your feet, relax your shoulders, relax your facial muscles and so on. Don't be afraid to become creative with these instructions and any others throughout the exercises. Remember you are in control. Your arm is becoming heavier and heavier. This will happen for two reasons, firstly because of the suggestion you are giving yourself that your arm will become heavier and heavier and secondly, it is physically difficult to hold your arm out at 45 degrees for extended periods of time. Lower your arm (resisting its downward movement) to your lap over a five-minute period. Then repeat with your other arm. *Each time your arms reach your lap you will feel a relaxation serge run throughout your entire body.* As you progress successfully into this stage of the exercise, your eyelashes may begin to flicker. This is the only way a beginner can confirm an altered state of consciousness brain wave pattern has been achieved. This exercise is very simple and if the flickering of eyelashes is not achieved on your first attempt, keep practising. However, some individuals may not experience flickering eyelashes. Towards the end of your arm lowering, count down from 40, imagine your favourite colour, suggesting to yourself, 'relax, relax, relax, I am becoming more and more relaxed.' The final part of the countdown is very important. When the count gets to zero, it is at this point, at this special window, we say our suggestion/affirmation. It is said mechanically and only once. e.g., *'54321 I am a happy, relaxed, strong individual with a high self-esteem.'* Immediately after saying your affirmation follow up with a visualisation, a positive daydream of your design. Many can actually see mind pictures in colour or black and white. If you cannot, then just imagine a picture.

In your mind's eye see yourself, for example, confident and relaxed in a social setting or imagine yourself walking down the street confident, respecting other individuals and being respected by them. You may visualise yourself sitting on a cosy sofa with your arms wrapped around yourself, feeling a warm loving feeling for yourself.

Remember, getting into a deep relaxed state is only a matter of practice. Tailoring making your own suggestions/affirmations and visualisations or daydreams are the key to your success. The most important thing to remember is consistency and perseverance – this means every day with heart, strength and conviction. It is so easy.

We will now look at how you can simply construct a simple program to improve and balance yourself as a person, and to improve or balance your self-esteem. The affirmations you use are positively constructed, by yourself, from a list of attributes you want to become your reality.

Before we can do this, you need to list the problem areas about yourself that you want to change. The following list demonstrates some examples:

List of Problems	List of the New Me
Lack of Humour	Humorous
Stressed	Relaxed
Lack of Confidence	Confident
Insecure	Secure
Angry	Rational/Assertive
Jealous	Secure
Sad	Happy
Fearful	Accepting/Rational

The following is a list of positive attributes that you may want to enhance:

Positive Enhancements	
Perfectionist	Balanced
Satisfied	Gratitude
Aggressive	Assertive
Happy	Contentment

When constructing affirmations keep them short, concise with no duplications. Place the most important messages first, always in the here and now and with the sense of having been already achieved – 'I am …'

Sample affirmation

'I am a relaxed, humorous, confident, rational and positive person who is tolerant, secure and happy'.

You are now in control. This is an example of an affirmation you could use in your relaxation exercise *at the end of the countdown*. It is interesting to note at this point that, down the track, as you are beginning to see change taking place, the affirmation can be altered and new words inserted, or some taken out. For example: You may have succeeded in uncovering/developing your sense of humour and consider taking the word humorous out of the affirmation and say, include the need to become more individual. The start of the affirmation would then read: 'I am a relaxed individual, confident, rational ...'

Once the desired attributes are established and the affirmation is constructed, you then create your own visualisations. A visualisation is simply a day-dream/state of mind that you construct and saturate your mind with, whilst the manipulative ego is 'asleep' when you are in a deep relaxed state. It is interesting to consider how often we send potent negative messages into our mind.

Remember you are the architect; you are in control because you can know yourself better than anybody else in this world.

As we have seen the affirmation is stated, only once, at zero after the countdown. You then introduce your visualisations/positive daydreams through your mind's-eye or imagine them on the TV screen in your mind.

Here are several examples of visualisations, but remember each of us are very different and the life experiences for another person would not necessarily apply to you.

Example 1: Confidence Building

You see yourself confidently walking into a room full of people. You move around confidently talking to each person. The people you speak to are interested in what you have to say and you are listening intently and genuinely to what they are telling you about themselves. You are liked and you like the communication you are experiencing.

Example 2: Liking Myself

You are seated in a quiet, cosy room on a soft carpet. You wrap your arms around yourself and feel love for yourself.

Example 3: Relaxation

You are sitting in a forest. You are relaxed and feeling one with nature. (Remember, if you had a bad experience in a forest, this visualisation would have to be constructed differently.) You can hear a breeze in the trees. You can feel the filtered sun on your face, you can smell the leaves, earth and moisture. You touch the earth and soil. You are completely relaxed.

You will find when stress manifests, as it does, if you practice your relaxation visualisation exercise, it will always be with you.

So just to recap:

1. Start the relaxation exercise.
2. Count down from forty. Tell yourself to relax Individual parts of your body. I am becoming more and more relaxed …
3. When you reach zero, say your affirmation once only, clearly and precisely.
4. Introduce two/four visualisations which you have prepared and add feeling for added impact and absorption.

If visualisations and affirmations can be experienced with feeling as well, the effect can be even more powerful. Here are two examples: If you are visualising strength, generate that strong feeling from chest, forehead or solar plexus. A feeling of happiness can be experienced in your heart, chest or solar plexus. We all have different areas of the body where we experience feelings.

With anything in life, persistence and patience is paramount. The preventative healing abilities of our unconscious can be trusted. Many of the behaviours and habits we have developed and those passed on from previous generations, will in time be replaced by the real you.

Who you really are will move slowly, but surely from within to balance the foxy and threatening ways of the ego.

Chapter 5

Dreams

Nightmares, Soul, Feelings, Precognition or All

Have you ever had the feeling that your life is being guided from somewhere else? We have spoken about the influence that our ego, our self-centred 'I, me and my' has over our behaviours, but could there be a bigger force at work deep in our psyche? A force constantly available, constantly updating and exclusively your very own. Your dreams.

Have you ever had a dream you felt was trying to tell you something? Been in a place before? Felt you could write a poem or paint something special? Felt an affinity with the wonders of the universe and earth's nature? Felt the wonders of the child within? Sensed a higher self, deep inside?

It's evident throughout all cultures that a force, a truth, emanates from deep inside their communal psyches giving positive cross generational guidance at the individual level.

It may be the great religions of the world, the Australian Aboriginal dreamtime, Native American spirituality, African indigenous religions and many more.

These experiences occur collectively worldwide, at national levels, within groups and at the individual level. However, we can all experience this magic originating from within.

A small boy walked into my room, stood beside my bed and looked straight up at me. I was sitting reading and in a half sleep state. What happened next was not a miraculous vision, but simply a visualization I was having in a part meditation, dream state.

The boy had a mop of blonde hair with a double crown at the top. Four to five years of age, he gazed up at me with large blue eyes, strong, but lost and lonely. I placed my hand on his shoulder and said to him, 'I know you are sad, but you are so brave and strong. I know you have been sick since you were a baby and your daddy has just come back from the war. You don't see daddy when you wake up because he has gone to work. Sometimes it's dark when he comes home so he can't play with you. He is very tired. He does love you, and so do I, very, very much. I play all the games you play, with my children and their children. Your mud pies, shops, paper aeroplanes and drawing with chalk on paths. They like playing in water, too.'

'I am here whenever you want to play or speak to me.' My hand moves to rest on his shoulder. 'There are very special people around you who love you and care for you. You know who they are and you will never forget them. Your mother is always here.'

Thank you, little man, for the love and bravery you have shown me. I have tried all my life to honour your struggle. I sometimes tried too hard, but we both know why, don't we?

The little boy is myself. My small child, within.

Our dreams have all types of functions, in the above case this visualization/active meditation allowed me to speak with the little boy within me, reassure him, show him the love his sensitivity perceived he was not receiving and share another love that each of us completely understand.

The visualisation/daydream allowed me to experience feelings dormant inside me for many years, understand the feelings, vent them and heal even more. This is an example of how perceived negatives and real negatives can be revisited and turned to a positive outcome.

(l deal with transmuting negative feelings and energies to positive in previous and later chapters).

Dreams do not happen by chance. There are many layers within the unconscious; dreams clearly show us this. Some dreams tend to deal with day-to-day experiences portraying conflicts, pent up feelings and fears that are sitting in the back of our minds. Simple dreams that portray daily conflicts we may think about, and throw off as we shower, but there are other dreams that stay with us for days, weeks and years. Some that tell us the future (precognitive dreams) and there are a few deep magic dreams that we never forget.

Then there are nightmares. Even those are explainable and helpful unless perverted by dietary or chemical influences.

Without any warnings, during sleep or daydreams (half sleep or meditation states), energies that have been pushed into our unconscious can be triggered back by the subtlest of thoughts, situations, music, aromas and places.

One of the tricks the unconscious mind uses, when we are awake or asleep, is called projection. Our unconscious, incredibly creates characters and situations and sagas in order to show us things we may not want to look at, or we are oblivious to, whilst our 'l, me and my', or our façade, is in control. Sleep lets our mind drop its guard and the magic of the unconscious creates the most incredible scenarios. We may dream of friends, adversaries or significant others such as movie stars, spiritual individuals, artists, musicians and see them in positive or negative ways. For example, we may dream of our best friend or lover and endow them with our deepest, finest qualities, be these real or imagined, to find later our expectations were way over the top. Some aspects of falling into the 'madness' of love can demonstrate dramatically how placing the highest imagined qualities of ourselves onto another can feel glorious, but when the true aspects of love, such as empathy, patience, unselfishness or kindness are not present, somebody always gets hurt.

A dream was told to me by a young man in his twenties. He had painted his lover all over in gold. His dream was telling him he had endowed her with qualities she did not possess, qualities he only aspired to from his own 'higher self or wishful perceptions'.

We may dream of a person we don't like and the unconscious will attempt to show us, through their negative behaviour, in the dream, the same faults that exist within our own character. 'That horrible Jackie is selfish and always tries to cause trouble talking about others'. What could be happening here is the unconscious is using the character Jackie to show you aspects of yourself that you are consciously unaware of, but have pushed to the back of your mind. We have to be careful here, for in order to get its point across, the unconscious can tend to accentuate, especially if you are oversensitive, dramatic and take things too seriously. Alcohol, chemicals, some foods and the onset of disease or virus can also accentuate dreams out of proportion.

There are some dreams of a deeper nature, sometimes referred to as precognitive. – (Jung,

1963). These dreams can appear to, in some cases, predict future events. This is quite possible, for if our unconscious is not directly affected by our wakening 'I, me and my' state, then a more objective view of future events is not out of the question. This can also be brought on purposely or just occur naturally when the ego is bypassed during meditation. Decisions, dreams and thoughts which are not influenced by our self/selfish persona or mask give an interpretation of ourselves, others and life, which can be more balanced and way ahead of the moment. Some may refer to this as psychic. For example, we may have a certain habit which we know deep down is not good for our well-being. A dream or a set of recurring dreams may, by way of an internal mini drama, show us the consequences of our negative behaviour using friends or invented characters which our mind uses or projects to, to get its message across. If we can learn to understand the messages in dreams, we can use them to give us our own personal cross-checks on our shortcomings and equilibrium, our highest potentials and creativity.

Every now and then a special dream can come along, a dream which may portray very deep and profound aspects of our life. An example of this type of dream will be covered later in this chapter.

The Australian Aboriginal Dreamtime dreams are also a good example of this. Dreams of individual members of tribes, over many thousands of years, have clearly set and established evolved rules and myths to live by. The spiritual aspirations of one of the oldest races on earth are passed on from one generation to the next by storytelling, dance and rock paintings.

Sleep time is where our unconscious can speak to us in a most precise, most beautiful and sometimes scary way. It would seem we can't have pleasant dreams without nightmares. But, is this not the way of the world and the universe?

It is a proven scientific fact that we all dream, although some would protest they do not, or if they do, they don't remember them. Placing a pad and pencil beside your bed and giving yourself the suggestion that you will recall your dreams, can be all it takes to remember them.

Does it matter if we dream or not? Apart from REM sleep, the state of sleep responsible for the restoration of the brain, can we gain anything from studying our dreams? Can dreams tell us anything or are they just meaningless prattle our minds make up? Do dreams vary in their nature? Are they sometimes passive, informative, problem solving? Are there dreams that warn of impending dangers, alert us to the complicity or the love of others? Can dreams inspire? Can they have some spiritual content? Can they cross time and take us back and give us a chance to re-look at the past or transport us into the future and show us what may take place? The answer to all these questions is, possibly, yes.

In the end, the most important thing about dreams is they are yours and yours alone. The symbols and the themes are like your fingerprints and your appearance, uniquely yours.

Is there anything to be gained by recording and studying our dreams and the unconscious? The answer to this question is, only if you have the need to delve into that mysterious, yet very normal, part of yourself.

Our unconscious communicates specific messages to us through dreams. If we don't get the information the first time, dreams of the same theme will occur until we understand the meaning. It would seem the unconscious will not let us down. Even seemingly negative information can be put to positive use.

Much has been written about universal dream symbols. That water could signify a cleansing process or portray peaceful areas of the unconscious. A forest could symbolise peace and regeneration. If a woman had been raped or a man had fought a war in a forest a symbol of peace and relaxation would not apply. If a boy near drowned in an ocean it would not be remembered in the same way as a teenage girl who found her first love by the sea. Each of us have our own particular symbols or myths, some borrowed and some created by ourselves and always, some a work in progress.

Our symbols within are as complex as the millions of experiences we have been exposed to since birth and possibly the effects passed on by our ancestors. Eye colour and physical features are passed on. Predisposition to longevity and certain illnesses we know are inherited. Varying temperaments in babies are noticeable not long after birth. It has been established that energies can also be genetically passed on from one generation to the next. A bird was not present when its nest was being built, how does it know how to construct a nest identically?

Your symbols, your own personal myths, are your very own, your own creation from billions of individual inputs and your very precise key to what lies deep within.

At this point, here is a simple example of a series of dreams demonstrating how we can use hidden personal messages deep within ourselves to identify a problem, act and change outcomes for the future. This dream clearly shows how the unconscious can, through dreams, keep sending us recurring messages until we understand. The saying, 'the answer was there all the time,' is so clear here.

The following set of dreams show the dreamer, conflict in her life, identification of her problem, resolution and the developing future. A woman in her thirties, let's call her Sally, has a series of recurring dreams leaving her feeling threatened, insecure and demonstrating she is not in control of her life.

She is on an underground train alone and the driver is travelling too fast and missing stations. In another dream she is going home and is seated at the back of a bus. Again the driver is driving dangerously, running red lights and missing stops. The next dream she is in a taxi and the driver is not listening to her directions.

All of these dreams kept recurring. When she accepted the unconscious was trying to tell her something, she realised her life was being controlled. She immediately told me her ex-partner was still ruling her life from a distance. The night before she had a different dream, she was riding a bicycle, it was unsteady and she had no brakes. After checking her personal symbols with her it was discovered her bicycle ride was her symbol of her new shaky independence. She was beginning to break away, in her mind, from her domineering ex-partner; riding the bicycle she now had control of her transportation and her life, albeit very shaky. After understanding those very definite messages put to her through dreams from her unconscious, she understood she now had choices: eliminate this person completely from her life, or be more assertive and retain him as a friend. She also realised that the kindness she showed to him was taken advantage of.

A young man, in his twenties, told me of a dream. This dream had a profound effect on him. It appears to display higher aspirations in both his current life and into the future.

He was in a steel-mesh capsule, with a mysterious long white-bearded oriental man. The cage lifted high into the sky above the most beautiful mountain range he had ever seen. The air was crisp and cool and he felt a tremendous feeling of peace and well-being, one with everything. In an instant his guide disappeared and the capsule went into free-fall. He thought he was crashing to his death, but the cage slowed as it neared the ground. He landed in a beautiful valley at the base of the majestic mountain range. He knew someday, he would have to climb to the top of that mountain and he knew he was not alone. This dream showed him incredible beauty and it showed he was being guided from within, but it also showed clearly attainment of peace and reaching lofty areas of the mind had to be earned by him and him alone — there are no free rides. These symbols and this story are his and his alone. It is his own small story, his own personal experience, just as your dreams are yours. This dream could be an example of a precognitive dream. An interpretation could be:

The oriental wise man may have been a character projected forwarded by the dreamer's unconscious mind — his higher self. In the soaring capsule, way above the mountain peaks, the dreamer was allowed to have a glimpse of higher levels of his consciousness. Returning to the beautiful valley, his climb could begin. The lift in consciousness, in the cage, only took seconds.

The spiritual mountain climb was to take a lifetime.

It is not unusual for all of us, at one time or another, to find ourselves lost and tangled up in negative situations, life's growing pains and seemingly unbearable personal conflicts. From most of life's negative experiences, growth and positives can emerge. The answer can always be found within.

The following reading is my own personal dream and demonstrates how a dream from a deep level within the psyche can describe, map out and predict future perceptions and realities.

My dream as set out in my book *Fine Line* is included as part of my fictional character Geoffrey Blake's experience.

There is a degree of self-indulgence describing the following experience. I present the following with humility to document an actual experience of the depth of the psyche.

... Loud roars and howls from behind two huge oak doors stop me in my tracks. I am curious, my chest is tightening, my heart is beginning to pound. I must look inside. Pressing my fingers between the

two massive doors. I steadily push until they begin to open.

In my dream all is silent as I slide open the warehouse doors. I'm scared, but I must go in. Before me, a narrow cobble stone path disappears into the musky dinginess of the old building. I move inside, the doors close by themselves leaving me temporarily blinded.

From my right comes an excruciating, trumpeting screeching sound, which echoes around the whole building. I stand – I can't move – my heart is racing. Then out of the gloom I'm hit by a massive blow to my mid-section. I buckle over. A second blow throws me to the floor. A small, elephant-like animal with long, curled, thin ivory tusks, swipes at me for the third time, but a restraining chain holds the angry animal back. Another agonizing cry cuts through the air as the longhaired elephant's huge tusks catch my leg and spin me around on the stone floor.

It's not too late, I can still go back ... no, I say to myself, I must go on. I have no choice; I must see what is inside.

Suddenly from a stone pen on my left, a massive crocodile attacks with open jaws. I roll away as an iron grate stops this evil reptile's assault.

I feel if I keep in the centre of the path I will be safe. If I move too far either way, I will be done for.

Covered in animal excreta, mud and rancid water, I crawl on my hands and knees.

Bats and pigeons flutter about in the half-light. Huge pythons lie on rocks, and hang motionless only inches away from me. Apes and monkeys are swinging and screeching, the larger animals menacing the small. A usually harmless, long-armed sloth comes threateningly close to me, curls its upper lip, stares and hisses at me.

Seals and penguins hideously packed into a small rock-pool enclosure are all trying to survive together in putrid conditions. A fairy penguin lies crushed by a frustrated, snorting bull sea lion.

I stand and move on past these dismal pens of aggravated and hopeless creatures. Stopping, I see a pathetic figure approaching, unrestrained, out of the gloom. As it gets closer, I know it's a male. He's stooped and walking side on. He takes a full step with his left foot and a half with the right; his uneven gait makes him look frightening. But I have no fear. I refrain from moving closer for I sense he is territorial. This creature in my dream is powerful, but has no pride. He seems ashamed of his own existence. As he crosses my path he glances quickly at me – he knows me. Slowly this grotesque, sad figure moves away into the gloom on his predetermined journey. I need to go no further.

Outside a small, silent, lifeless crowd is filing along a meandering walkway towards a wooden pavilion, on a hill in the distance. I join the queue of these characterless, expressionless people.

Inside the wooden pavilion on the hill, I can see a large square open area. An ancient man crouching in a locked steel cage. From all sides he is being viciously ridiculed and harangued by a crowd. They jab and aggravate the ancient man with sticks and iron bars. The saliva of children drips from the body hair of the wretched creature. His head is swaying back and forth, his questioning eyes sheltered by one hand, the other making futile attempts to fend off the attacks.

There is an overwhelming atmosphere of hate and fear as I climb a wooden staircase to a balcony overlooking the whole painful scene. The tormented caged man looks up at me, our eyes lock in a mutual stare. He cannot contain his anguish any longer and lets out two shrilled screams which echo around and around the pavilion. The crowd freezes and is instantly silent. Tears stream from my eyes. God, I can feel the condemnation of the crowd, I know that lonely feeling I feel like that hairy ugly creature.

After his venting screams, the ancient man relaxes – the crowd vanishes.

Here is my short and concise interpretation of my dream – my perception and understanding my own personal symbols:

The large warehouse doors opening symbolises me entering the unconscious state.

The cobble stone path down the centre of the warehouse is a symbol of the centre path through life or time.

The confined, aggravated animals representing my projected conditions of life at the physical level.

If I stray off the centre path I have angry confined energies of life, represented by the aggravated animals to contend with.

The light in the distance, hope or dreams or just light. The cross of the cobblestone paths, exactly what it seems. The path down the centre, the path of aspirations, the path of life. The path crossing from where the instinctive Neanderthal appears and crosses my path could represent the instinctive part of myself crossing my life's aspirational path.

The caged ape-man in the pavilion on the hill may represent my restrained instinctive me, ridiculed by the ignorant crowd which may be projections representing aspects of my confining personality, superego and over compensation from bigotry surrounding me as a child.

I stand up on the balcony overlooking all the turmoil and feeling genuine compassion for my own caged instinctive self. The Neanderthal and my higher self-making a mutual, empathic connection.

One dream seems to contain a life's endeavours and aspirations. But again, only my perceptions, feelings and personal symbols.

Our personal perceptions and feelings may not be the actual reality, but apart from the judgments of others, and the releasing of karma, that is all we have.

The higher self is always aware of the truth. We only need to open the door.

Dreams can assist us by showing us both negative and positive, how they complement, helping us to understand what is stored deep in our unconscious.

Chapter
6

My Personal Myths
What is Your Personal Myth?

Often, we try to make sense of life, understand its opposing forces, nature, and the universe. This has been going on ever since people have been evolving and inhabiting the earth. We know this through cave paintings, early architecture, transcripts, folklore, song, art and literature. The essence of communal and individual lives' myths have been recorded, in both practical and unconscious ways, passing down through the ages.

What do you burn to do in this life, with its many stages of change? Again, the ego can have us engaged in following energies that our hearts and minds are duped into believing are real to us. We are, most times, held down by forces and energies we yearn to transcend; our calculating subjective self in firm, subtle control. Where does that leave us? Wasting valuable time? We can stumble through life with glimmers of what we are about, or we can conscientiously find out what makes us tick at the individual level, and go for it.

Who am I? What do I really want? What do I excel at? What motivates me? If we don't tick these boxes, what is the point and how does this vacuum affect our physical health, psychological health and subsequently, those around us?

So much more blinds us from finding our real selves than we realise. We are influenced from the day we are born by a myriad of outside forces and energies. Experiences of previous generations and genetic predispositions are passed onto us. In the first few years of our lives, we begin to model the behaviours and influences of our parents, significant others and community. We are constantly bombarded and influenced by so many things without realising.

It is important to understand what personally moves and motivates us. Once we identify our deep personal motivating forces, the meaning of our life intensifies with focus, interest and boundless energies.

What is your personal myth or myths? Deep inside we are all intuitively aware of what fires us up. Should we feel we have failed if we are bogged down and blinkered? – No, because it is a normal condition which can be transmuted to an 'enjoyable' and exciting process of release and growth. Wouldn't it be great to be doing what makes you feel good and get paid for it? If you do what you love, you will do it so well. If you love children, work with them. If you want to study music or singing, go for it. Work in agriculture, with the underprivileged, adventure and travel, the sciences; you possibly have many inner personal myths varying in intensity, overlapping, ebbing and flowing, still being discovered. The important thing is to, through the higher faculties of your mind, let blossom what really motivates you.

If the search for truth and balance within is a basic driver in your life, many entrenched habits and behaviours will surface, once challenged, to maintain their egocentric dominance. The more we progress, the more cunning and determined our self-impulses focus and intensify.

If aspiring to discover the various segmented stages or lives we experience in the years we are allotted, a mentor may be required. A true mentor will be a reflection and consolidator of your most inner potentials with little reliance on human doctrines or creeds. Conversely, the affirmations of organised groups, especially from those that promote fear as a means to personal growth and enlightenment, merely postpone the process of individuality. The myth of Jesus Christ being a strident example of a person who moved on from the teachings of the Essenes and followed a path of individuality, living by example and not personally recording any of his teachings.

Balance and answers to complex life situations can be accessed through active meditation, prayer, the arts, discipline, trust and guts, not always through the rigidity of the intellect which can be invariably influenced by the persistent, ruthless ego.

It is felt by many that the ego, the higher self and the intellect can work together on the path to individualisation. They can and do, but only in the intermediary stages of higher individual development. Most of us, however, have to contend with life or many of our lives in one, where there is constant to-ing and fro-ing between the intellect, the perceptions of the self and the higher self, which are constantly conflicting. This constraint, this distraction holds us to ordinary time. There are other dimensions and time zones where individuality, creativity, expanded consciousness and peace of mind accelerate and lift to undreamed of levels.

It may be our myth, or one of our many myths, to transcend this merry-go-round and release the imprisoned splendour. Understanding the intellect, the ego and their incredible ability to hold us captive is only the first step. Discipline and communication with the higher self, with trust, unwinds this complex triad. However, the more we trust and balance, the more cunning, in conjunction with the intellect, the ego and the superego can become, especially where high sensitivity within an individual is involved.

What does the real you want? It's a simple question and the answers are constantly within providing we are motivated to seek. It's a 'gentle' constant coming home.

The magical movie, 'The Wizard of Oz' sums it up through its perfectly generated characters, representing all aspects of its main character Dorothy's conscious and unconscious journey.

- Due to the complex perceptions of the author and the individual interpretations of those who love the story, it would contravene my belief in the personal uniqueness of each individual's myths and symbols to deeply analyse all characters, although at a very deep level I understood it all as a small child and to this very day I still identify with it, in its entirety. The continuing impact and appeal that The Wizard of Oz has over the generations attests to many common mythical denominators the story exquisitely projects. Dorothy's ego, symbolised by the lion, tinman and the scarecrow made of straw, make the journey together, along the Yellow Brick Road to meet the wizard, her alter ego. Against a background of positive and negative energies, symbolised by the wicked witch of the west and the good

witch of the north, she understands
the manipulations of the Wizard and
returns to the higher realms of her
mind, represented by simply coming
home.

It is a perfect example of how perceptions initiated by the self can lead one on a meandering, yellow brick path. The ego plays and fights for time. The higher realms and the higher self are timeless. The physical body is caught in the middle of these personal evolutionary processes, but protected by the healing influences of the higher self.

There is no place like home – home within, which is and always been there.

Chapter 7

The Blues

It is difficult for most of us to recognise whether our mood levels are affected by our immediate situations, the egos of others, past environments, previous ancestral influences, or deeper archetypal common denominators – the big movers (see chapter 11 The Big Movers) or a fluctuating cocktail of all. To identify the influences, to watch their interaction, to isolate them and their hideous, complex, combined impenetrable wall is the challenge.

The practical information in this chapter came about as a result of my personal search for a procedure to analyse and modify the complicated contributing factors which make up a depressed state or blue moods.

Advice can suggest we meditate, go into hypnosis, pray, keep busy, stay present. But as we all know when that 'blue' state comes along, it seems to have a way of its own. Besides, it is advised by the experts that going into a hypnotic state or dwelling on negatives, whilst depressed can in fact aggravate a depressed condition. As with many human conditions, where possible, prevention is far better than cure. But sometimes, even achieved balance can be rocked by an alignment of negative energies.

We all have the ability to soar to great heights in our minds, but we also have the same ability to plunge to the depths. Maintaining a middle path between the opposites in this life is becoming more and more difficult as the world shrinks with technology and the explosion in population. Streams of negative news are beamed instantaneously, from all over our planet, to us, hourly. If we had settlements on the moon or Mars, as we will soon, news will stream back and forth from there also.

What do we do with negative thoughts that originate from within and those projected at us by the world and other minds? We can pretend they don't exist, but when we push them away to the back of our minds, we tend to give them energy and out they pop out again, sometimes with more power than before. If we work hard, take alcohol, become involved in conflict, shop or rely on material things to distract us; that may work for a while.

When enough of these negative messages from within and outside swamp us we can become fearful, overwhelmed, exhausted, scared, disoriented and confused for short or long periods of time

Those that have experienced the demoralising effects of depression can understand how difficult it is to deal with. For friends and family looking on it can be a nightmare of helplessness, that is, if they realise. The type of depression I am speaking about here is not caused by physical health problems, deep psychological problems, and disease or chemical imbalances although, however, if present, they will be huge complicating factors. What I am referring to here are the blues, day to week, human confusions and fears, general stress caused by modern living, the stimulus of the media and the press, negative or perceived negative influences from our present, near present, our childhood, all clustering together to lower our spirits. Fears of current and future health problems, our mortality, not performing as well as we perceive we should, or not always getting what our ego wants, when it wants it.

Sometimes the origin of these bouts cannot be identified and actually be added to by dreams we can or can't recall. If we can move outside the influence of our 'I, me and my' we can begin to see situations from a more global, objective point of view. This is where negatives can in fact be turned to positives and where the silver linings of our lives start to flash through from deep within into our conscious state.

It is not the aim of the following exercises to replace professional help, but to empower an individual to do something for themselves, in those early hours of the morning and in those times in your life when you are 'on your own'.

The following very simple exercise can ease and help cure the paralysing condition of the blues which can take hold of any of us for hours, days, even years. Sensitivity in an individual can be an asset, but sometimes aggravate depression. The intellect and spiritually can sometimes be powerless to turn negativity around in the short term once it takes its tight grip.

The lack of correct food, sleep and exercise and the use of alcohol and drugs take us further away from peace of mind. Sugar being one of the main contributors to mood swings. Prescribed drugs can be effective, but the side effects should be noted. All drug side effects are well listed on Google.

We could visualise depression/the blues as a spinning grey ball of many interacting situations, problems and energies, imaginary and real, spinning out of control, getting larger, closer knitted and continually gathering more and more momentum and strength.

During various stages of this downward, tightening spiral we sometimes muster the energy to approach this spinning grey ball to try to slow its relentless overpowering hold on us.

With momentary enthusiasm we approach the grey mass armed with understanding, reason, the best hope we can muster, just to be thrown back feeling helpless again with nowhere to turn.

There is a way to slow this self-perpetuating grey spinning ball, that baron blackness. We need to pull it apart, unravel it and see it for what it really is: a conglomeration of reinforcing fears, misconceptions, mixed perceptions, misunderstandings all bound up with temporary lost hope. Once unravelled each life situation can be dissected and assessed. Its part in your temporary darkness can be monitored and dealt with separately. The insidious power this state of mine relies on is the ever changing, grouping together of seeming negatives and their daily, hour to hour, constantly varying and ever-changing combinations. It's like trying to play soccer with many goal posts that are continually being moved around.

What we perceive as negative feelings hurt, but even negative feelings can have positive outcomes. I often quote words from songs of the past. 'Try To Remember' is a song by Harvey Schmidt from the 40's. 'Without the hurt the heart is hollow.'

Below is set out a simple, original, tried and tested procedure which puts you slowly, but surely back in balanced control of the blues/depression. This procedure can be used to deal with past and future situations before they take hold. Even today there is indecision amongst psychodynamic and behavioural professionals whether we should delve into the past for answers (the psychodynamics) or alter our behaviours (the behaviourists) in the here and now. What I present is a combination of both psychodynamic and behavioural approaches. The psychodynamic approach looks into the past, at circumstances, situations of individuals, or groups that have influenced your present state. The behavioural approach basically ignores the past and deals with the here and now behaviours.

Let's get started:

Take a pen and list all the things that worry you. These can be financial, family (immediate and past generations) work, health, relationships, friendships, the future, the past, aspects of your childhood, your home. List individual people and make a split detailed break-up of differences and conflicts which may exist. Also list all the positives happening in your life. This can also include past positives that flow into the present. You can also list dreams and motivations into the future. This list will form the basis of our spreadsheet and can be added to or items removed as situations cease to be a worry for you.

This is the first step, the identification and breaking up of all aspects of your life that give degrees of concern over a specific time frame. We will then include a list of all the 'positives' that are happening for you at present and grade them also. Included in the positives are expressions of gratitude, future dreams and inspirations.

The aim of this approach is not to replace our ongoing endeavour to live in the here and now. This is your specific invitation to invite seeming negatives and seeming positives into your spotlight and note what they are and expose their interaction. It's your perceptions (our 'I, me and my') of what the 'lows' and 'highs' are, their ever changing, combined effect that causes confusion, which in many cases is just what the negative illusive ego thrives on.

We are by no means trying to focus on negatives. We are inviting positives and negatives into our conscious state, putting them under the magnifying glass in a disciplined way, observing the interaction we take away their power over us.

It is a flowing system. As some of your listed problems or momentary highs come into balance, they can be eliminated and new positives and negatives inserted.

There are problems and situations in life, which are not meant to be changed by our reasoning, perceptions or efforts. Once we come to the realisation something cannot be changed, we have no other alternative other than to accept and move on. The process of acceptance is difficult to arrive at through the guidance of the ego. How each of us connects to the higher faculties of our minds is an individual process. These entries that appear on our spreadsheet as consistently high negative scores, once accepted, can be reduced back to a score of say 1 with the letter A for acceptance in the same box. Keep them listed, because even accepted situations can change.

I once showed my son my personal spreadsheet indicating to him that I had a handle on all the particular negative components in my life at that time. He said, 'That's great dad, but what are you going to do about these?' (Two of the recorded items). He pointed out, it's one thing to record stress, another to take assertive action and make some overdue decisions.

Note, as negatives decrease, be they real or perceptual, overall outlooks and scores can gather their own momentum towards balance.

Claire's Problems: Positives and Negatives

		1/10	2/10	3/10
Christie's (14-year-old daughter)				
	Asthma	+3	-5	-6
	School Pressure	-8	-6	-7
	General Health	+7	+3	+2
	Bullied at School	-4	-	-5
Best Friend				
	Breast Cancer	-7	-7	-7
	Marriage Problems	-8	-6	-3
Lachlan, husband				
	Temper	-6	-1	-
	Snoring	-3	-3	-2
	Spending	-6	-7	-5

	Helps Me	+7	+8	+9
	Limited Quality Time	-2	+6	+7
Mum				
	Intolerance	-3	-3	+3
	Health	-7	-6	-4
	Assistance to Me	+8	+8	+9
Car Accident				
	Damage	-6	-6	-4
	No Transport	-7	-8	-4
	Nobody Hurt	+8	+9	+9
My Health				
	Today General	+6	+7	+8
	Flat Feet	-2	-2	-1

	Sinus	-2	+3	+6
	Digestion/Heart Burn	-1	+2	+3
Brother's Drinking		-7	-7	-7
Finances				
	Credit Cards	-2	+2	-
	Car Rego	-3	-	-
	Bills	-2	-4	+4
	Budget – Up and Down	+2	+3	+5
My Dog Penny		+8	+8	+9
	Health	+7	+7	+6
Money Arguments		-5	+2	-
Childhood				
	Less Affection than Brother	-3	-3	-3

	Popular at School	+7	+7	+7
	Running – School Champ	+7	+5	+7
My Shape				
	Skinny Legs	-4	+2	+4
	Small Boobs	-5	-1	-
Lack of Confidence		+6	+8	+8
What I am Grateful For				
	My Health	+8	+8	+7
	My Marriage	+6	+7	+5
	My Children	+9	+9	+7
	Holidays Coming	+9	+9	+9
	My Friends	+6	+7	+4
World Pressures		-2	-4	+1

The Blues

	Trump	-9	-8	-9
	Constant Conflicts	-4	-4	-2
	World Childhood Conditions	-3	+1	-5
	World Population Growth	-1	-1	(-3) 1A
	Rights of Women	+2	+2	+3
	Global Warming	-	-2	-4
Australian Problems				
	Equal Pay for Women	+6	+6	+3
	Child Care	+5	+7	+4
	Refugees	-6	-4	-3
Intend to Take Singing Lessons		+7	+8	+9
Going Back to University		+8	+8	+8
	Totals	14	64	82

Michael's Problems: Positives and Negatives

		1/6	2/6	3/6
Finances				
	Credit Card	-8	-8	-9
	Super Going Down	-2	-	-
	House Payments	+2	+2	+2
	Interest Rate Rise	-5	-4	-5
Work				
	Staff Cuts	-7	-4	-3
	Work Load	-3	-2	-1
	Bigoted Manager	-6	-5	-7
	Promising Future	+3	+4	+1
	Love My Work	+5	+5	+5

	General Economics	-2	-2	-3
Ears Stick Out		-3	-3	-3
Wife (Jackie)				
	Early Menopause	-6	-7	-8
	Spending	-4	-2	-4
	Takes Advantage of My Good Side	-1	-	-2
	Love Her	+6	+6	+6
	Gall Bladder Operation	-2	-3	-1
	Jackie's Expectations	-4	-4	-4
	Jackie Flirts	-3	-3	-4
Buying a Boat		+6	-	+4
Upgrading to New Car		+3	+4	+4
Doing Well at Golf		+5	+5	+5

Living With the Other Side

Scott (Son, 19 Years Old)				
	Doing Well in Soccer	+4	+5	+5
	Will Not Listen	-5	-2	-5
	Alcohol	-4	-4	-5
	Driving Fast	-3	-3	-5
Jamie (Daughter 14 Years Old)				
	New Boyfriends	-7	-8	-4
	Star Netball Player	+4	+3	+4
	Will Not Listen	-3	-4	-6
	Comes Home Late	-2	-5	-7
Health				
	Wisdom Tooth	-7	-8	-4
	New Prescription Glasses	-5	-4	-1

The Blues

Love for Coffee		+4	+5	+5
AFL – Love the Game		+7	+8	+8
World Unrest		-3	-2	-2
House Renovations		+3	+6	+7
Brother (Lance)				
	Chain Smoker	-4	-2	-2
	Cheating on his Wife	-3	-3	-5
	Lance loved more than me when we were kids	-3	-4	-3
My Next Birthday is 50		-7	-7	(-8) 1A
Holidays next September		+7	+7	+8
Intend to Take Up Flying		+8	+8	+8
Thinking of Opening a Plant Nursery		+8	+9	+9
	Totals	-37	-26	-30

Chapter 8

Negative Energies, Positive Energies and Feelings

The symbiotic relationship between negative and positive energies (the opposites) has been going, in the universe, for billions of years. The conflicting and balancing of the opposites is a natural process which equalises our environment and the human psyche bringing out the best in our civilisations, albeit a slow and painful evolutionary process. Each one of us is constantly connected to cosmic energies, collective human energies, interpersonal and individual feelings and energies. The human psyche has the unique ability to create its own 'reality' leading to a myriad of complications, both constructive and destructive.

Day to day, at the personal level, we all experience the effects of negative energies. We also experience the effects of positive energies. We attempt to understand the effect negative and positive energies have on us. The opposing positive and negative energies are the constant reality, it is how we perceive negative and positive that is the variable.

Free will is an integral part of human growth, although many would disagree pressing their outdated perceptions, myths and gender bias. It is difficult for those wanting immediate change to be objective, for the pressure to change the world, in one lifetime, is, in many cases, crucial to the individual's ego or super ego's base.

Extremists in their haste, their insistence, their power, their 'know it all perceptions', in many cases exacerbate conflict through cultural prejudice and bias. Short term gullibility, across sections of the human population, is very vulnerable to those practicing projection, blame, misplaced ideals and self-centred manipulation. However, in time, even these negatives set the process of positive change in motion, painful as that may be. If we trust enough, the silver lining of acceptance begins to shine through.

Negative and positive energies can also enter our conscious minds as premeditated, or uncontrollable, compulsive thoughts and feelings (free floating thoughts or through abstract associations and inspirations) triggered by sounds, influence of others, smell, life situations, sight, competition, yearnings, greed, and infatuation. These energies are not necessarily linked to self-esteem, sensitivity or intelligence, however, low self-esteem or perceived low esteem, oversensitivity, perceptions of various intellects, and lack of empathy can aggravate feelings of negativity and fear. Natural hormonal, chemical imbalances in the body, disease and brain deterioration can accentuate outlooks and emotions, not to mention the effects of so-called recreational or prescribed drugs and alcohol.

The state of perceived happiness/bliss can also be taken for granted, idealised and distorted. It was once said to me, 'we know what we learn from pain and suffering, but what do we learn from 'happiness'?

Do we ever come to terms with our fears? Is it possible to find contentment and acceptance within the opposites? The answer is yes, we do it every day.

The conglomeration of negative and positive energies can originate from many sources:

1. Present day to day, hour to hour negative, or what we perceive to be negative actions, feelings and events.

2. Negative and positive actions from our past either instigated by ourselves or an individual or individuals that were in our past proximity.

3. Negative and positive tendencies from previous generations which have

directly passed on behaviours and genetic predispositions.

4. Negative and positive energies stemming from previous and current community influences.

5. Broader positive and negative cultural and folklore influences.

6. Worldwide negative and positive energies, current and back through history from genetics, passed down behaviours and thousands of organised religious influences.

7. The influence of the media and social technology, these days world-wide and instantaneous.

8. The influence of a friend.

9. The influence of animals, wild and pets.

10. Natural catastrophes on our planet and the threat of, say, asteroid damage from outer space, or threats from an unpredictable universe

Negative energies can take the form of feelings, emotions, actual confrontations with other individuals or groups, or uncontrollable free-floating anxieties. Abstract, imagined or real manifestations of 'positive' and 'negative' energy can sweep into our consciousness with no warning, being triggered by music, a movie, a smell, a place, relationships, past relationships, a single word or drugs and alcohol. Sometimes these negative energies, and positive energies, hit us from several sources at once (refer chapter 6) overwhelming us and, apart from performing various therapeutic exercises, all we can do is hang in there until they pass – as they mostly do. Many of our negative fears and thoughts actually turn out to be positive. These can be called 'happy endings.' 'Look for the silver lining when a cloud appears in the blue,' are the words of a popular Western song by Jerome Kern from the 1920's.

It would seem what we deem negative can sometimes have a positive outcome and what we call happiness can be quite the opposite. It is a fact that lottery winners very rarely find happiness as a result of their winnings. Some find 'happiness' in revenge, undermining another's self-esteem and other cruel practises.

How can we balance out the roller coaster ride when there is so much negativity around us, apart from what we may actually create for ourselves? The news reports tend to focus on shortcomings because peddlers of negative information are well aware there is an insatiable appetite for it.

The question is not why we are this way, but how can we change these predispositions. Flitting around the surface of negativity and trying to be positive helps, but does not change much. We need a consistent brave approach to understand fear and negative energies. All the great old religions of the world have similar solutions to combating the extremes of the psyche. But it is difficult to sustain the idea that one size fits all, because it does not. Even though there are common denominators, we are all individual and different. We need to have techniques and exercises which are transportable, specific, flexible, and are adjustable to our individual needs. (See chapter 4)

If negative is transmuted to positive and positive is negative, how can we tell the difference? How do we deal with these seeming positive and seeming negative messages that come from deep inside us? The first thing to remember is to consider what is negative and what is positive.

A negative message from our unconscious can in fact be a positive message in disguise and vice versa. This is very evident in some of our dreams. We must however, remember that dreams can dramatise and distort, and symbols in dreams are unique to the individual. (See chapter 5 Dreams) This could be the reason some organised religions are hot and cold when it comes to placing reliance on dreams as a personal, individual growth tool. However, the mythical history of most religions is to vigorously use dreams of its prophets as cornerstones of their faith. Prophetic dreams and visions are often referred to in the Hebrew bible. The Christian bible continually presents dreams and visions as a source of wisdom and predication. The very ancient tribes of Australia and of the deepest wildernesses of our planet rely on dreams as a basis of their mythology.

A neighbour once came to my door and explained, 'I had a dream last night that Hitler visited me at my house.'

The message in this dream seems obvious, or is it? His dream was giving him a message and the intensity of the symbols his psyche produced were showing him feelings he had pushed into the back of his mind. His brain had produced a picture and given him a seemingly negative message about himself, or did it? He could look at the dream this way. 'My deeper or higher self – my God level, is showing me that part of my approaches to my life are dictatorial, letting me realise that some aspects of Hitler's behaviour could apply to me. 'I am not a murderer, I love people, I am a positive father with five lovely children and a beautiful wife. But I should look at the part of myself which can be too forceful and have the need to manipulate.' He concluded. The message, although seeming negative, is positive.

Years later he contacted me and asked if I would like to visit the church of which he was now an elder.

Whenever we are plunged into conflicts with close ones, friendships or people generally, we may have a tendency to panic, blame, lash out, play the victim, bully, manipulate quietly, passively or loudly and aggressively.

There is a song, 'You Always Hurt the One You Love by Jimmy Roselli …. 'the one you love shouldn't hurt at all.' Other acquaintances usually suffer our *projections less. Times like this, although painful and sometimes devastating, can actually have positive aspects. Spontaneous venting of feelings, say, in a disagreement, can get feelings off the chest, being a disguised positive. Incredible seeming nastiness and even malice can freely flow forward, but it would seem an inner wise old owl understands. Forgiveness mostly blossoms forth? The *wise old owl* might say;

> 'This is only emotional.'
> 'Look up at the stars.'
> 'This will pass, all things do.'
> 'This will not be the end of your world.'
> 'See, you feel better now.'

*Faults or emotional bubble ups of our own blamed onto somebody else.

Now what about those negative feelings, energies or 'voices' that pop into our minds from nowhere? We all experience those. Where do they come from, how can they be stopped? Should they be stopped? When we become scared, feel sad, tired or maybe when it is wet and miserable out of doors is the ideal time for the heebie-jeebies to move into our mind. Some of us pray, some meditate. We might go to the movies or plan a holiday. Some attempt to stay in the moment – the here and now, talk things out with a trusted friend or see a counsellor. If we can trust tomorrow is another day and what worries us today may change completely. (Refer Chapter 6, The Blues.)

Deep-seated pains within individuals either from current life, or passed on behaviours or genetic predispositions from previous ancestral roots, can continually fuel these periodic outbursts of fear and pain, which subside and reappear time and time again. Sometimes negatives from the past and present can accidentally or purposely link together in a relentless temporary plunge downward.

Where do we get answers from within ourselves without the devastating, controlling, disruptive, destructive influence of the ego, our 'I, me, and my?' It is possible to obtain these answers and it can be achieved easily and quickly. It is referred to as active meditation. Simply finding the answers to complex situations by by-passing our ego. Many find prayer is another way of achieving objective answers from our higher self or 'God' consciousness. How often, planting a mind seed, have we slept on a problem after 'putting it out there' to find the answer materialises. 'Out there' being a popular expression, which gives credence to the idea that answers to complicated day to day questions can be obtained from areas of the psyche away from the influence of the ego (our 'I, me and my') or the intellectually educated mind. *Problem solving using Active meditation we have partially dealt with in Chapter 4.

At the family and community level there is a constant exchange of positive and negative perceptions and feelings backed by cultural mix, religions, ancestral genetics, male and female standpoints, sexual orientations, young, middle age groups, and older. Throw in political and big business interests and we have a very complicated mix. When God-consciousness aspirants, intellectuals and general selfishness collide, is it any wonder we end up confused? But all is not lost. If as an individual, we can stand back and trust that all this exchange of energies has a purpose and is in fact steadily on the way to positive, giving us a chance to grow. We can save ourselves a great deal of wasted time, energy and life if we sometimes just observe and trust in our inner and outer universe, albeit with its massive constant contrast. There are times, however, when we have to be fearless and assertive from a base of balance. There are also times when we hold on, grin and bear and soldier on.

The balance and evolution of the universe and our own individual selves is sometimes difficult to understand and accept, but we are children of the universe and acceptance is basically what life is about. If we as children of the universe have trouble with such an impersonal, vast concept, then it is understandable why some try to view their inner and outer universe by substituting human entities as paternal, human symbolic bridges. Many more get stuck in between rejecting the simplistic mythology of religion, and trusting the inevitability and complementary contrasts of an unpredictable, but magic universe we live in. On the broader spectrum mythology can offer us only limited resolution, for in the end acceptance is the common denominator. Mythology and religion may change the giving and taking realities of the psyche, but they cannot change the realities of the universe. If an earthquake is going to occur, there is nothing we can do to stop it. Some would believe God is to blame or should be expected to intervene. If an individual is spared from a natural catastrophe, it may only be the ego that would thank God.

Are seeming positive energies that come from within and from the outside actually negative or vice versa? How can we see through our perceptions and the perceptions of others? Can we do this from our ego, our 'I me and my', or does this ability to see through the fog come from another aspect of ourselves? If so, what area is that? An area of condemnation, idealism, rebellion, religion, the material, violence, escapism or intellectual humility, acknowledgement of all as brothers and sisters, the higher self within or the acceptance of the universe? There are many approaches.

Is it ok to have negative feelings? Feelings do not make the individual, positive or negative – one is as big an illusion as the other. Wow, that seems to leave a big blank space, or does it? Maybe that is where our real self exists.

It could be less devastating and a more peaceful transition if the swing of the pendulum, between our ego and our higher self was not so extreme. Modern day leaders such as Obama, Lincoln, Kennedy, Gandhi, and Martin Luther King, all constantly strived for non-violent, empathic, assertive progress. Over a multitude of generations to come these will be the individuals that will stand out and be remembered, not those who play to, and rise to power identifying and using fears, prejudices, negative perceptions and the potential aggressiveness of sections of the populace.

We trust in the fact that the sun is going to rise each morning, even though some days there will be clouds. Nature will continue to flourish, with or without us, one way or another, regardless of our interferences.

Throughout history many have tried to govern skilfully pandering to the masses. Great leaders over the last 2000 years and before, have demonstrated progress from a base of empathy and compassion. Deep within all of us is trust, empathy and compassion. But, there is a tendency for humans to short cut, usually with the assistance of the individual selfish aspects of the ego, or at the hands of leaders well versed in the art of manipulating us using blame, fear, racial prejudices, and isolationism.

Both forms of leadership are very compelling. Do they complement each other? In the process of ongoing evolution, individual's choosing a negative path will suffer stress. Stress which will eventually compromise the physical body. The same inner discord can result from over indulgences and the complacency of success.

Throughout history many have tried to govern attempting and unscrupulously projecting the negative perceptions of the masses, to find it is only possible to fool some of the people some of the time.

Sadly, even this opposite swing of human energies, the path of nonviolence, moves towards peace and the erupting from our fiery core, not unlike the planet we live on, appears to be necessary to balance the collective psyche.

Simply, our basic human instinct is survival and promotes a safe, constructive, accepted environment, a striving for an accepting, empathic balanced psyche, with gratitude, which is best for our children and our inner child.

Chapter
9

The Troll Under the Bridge

No matter how things progress in a positive way, the troll under the bridge is always lurking, in the shadows. Do the terrible trolls exist or are they just a mythical representation of something far deeper and sinister ever present in the human psyche?

What I am speaking about here is not the blues or depression, it is something very different. From time to time the gremlins and trolls march spontaneously forward from our unconscious state uninvited and create havoc. No matter what we do we cannot halt their advance. They dance their shadowy dances until partially vented, then retreat back into the dark spaces. If we repress them, they gain extra energy, lay dormant to reappear again and again. Are these shadowy figures real? (They seem real enough for us to give them various names and include them in most adult and children's stories, to embellish the plots.)

The universe has times of mayhem, times of peace, plateauing and times of spectacular progress. Each and every one of us is a micro-part of the universe and experiences its, and our own, complex menu of parallel complementary and opposite energies.

Let's focus on the 'dark grey area', these short, but potent, periods of unusual darkness, I refer to as 'the invasion of consciousness' by the shadowy dark trolling aspects of the unconscious. These can move in at any time, as can enlightened invasions of the conscious mind by unconscious content. Some might say, when enlightened moments occur, we are visited by angels.

The source of these shadows can come from many levels of our unconscious minds, triggered by the energies from our immediate past, our individual ancestral history, communal history or a wider collective of accumulated human experiences. Sometimes they can manifest as individual and separate forays or they can group together and invade our consciousness as a massive combined outpouring, commencing with one theme pulling other shadowy themes in as momentum is gained.

Not all the shadowy stuff comes directly from our own relatively short lifetime of experiences. We know energies, negative and positive, are passed on from previous generations. Apart from the physical hand me downs such as storytelling, writing, music, painting and now the internet, we are still learning scientifically about genetics, cultural influences and worldwide collective unconsciousness.

Let's take an example. Something may be upsetting us at the daily level, combine this with troubles from our relatively short existence, some negative predispositions passed on from our previous generations, plus some cultural norms and then add some collective world problems past and present. A 'perfect' storm. No wonder we get confused and fearful. The reverse can happen, good stuff from all these levels can align and we can feel incredible. Both extremes need to be monitored. A combination of positive and negative can also be difficult to fathom and navigate. Refer to chapter 6, The Blues.

Birds and animals migrate without being shown, the information is passed through their generations from way, way back. What we are exposed to in the womb and whilst we are very young, what we repress as children as the result of treatment at the hands of older children and adults, can add to these shadows, both realistically and unrealistically. Situations and circumstances also add to positive and negative experiences. Due to our perceptions, our memory and our imagination, events can be distorted. Shadows we create as our egos grow and we become adults, all sit back there in the back recesses of our minds with a need to come forward through dreams, emotional venting, fantasy, free floating anxieties and inspirations, naturally come forward and subsequently balance out. However, we tend to push the negatives back and inadvertently increase their future momentum.

Shadowy figures and related scenarios form a great deal of dream content and can become highly accentuated, stylised and out of proportion. So, we must be careful not to overreact here. I am not referring to criminal behaviour or the sad realities of atrocities that have occurred throughout history, or the physical damage that occurs currently minute by minute throughout the world. Sadly, their combinative effect does play a big part. What I am referring to is negative energies, sometimes obvious and sometimes only abstract or symbolic. Do we fight or trust? Do we have control over what happens in the extremities of our minds? Repressing these shadowy events or ignoring them is only going to accentuate their power.

As a five-year-old I would go to bed fearing those horrible nightmares that would return again and again. Reassurances from mum and dad, not to think about them and they would go away, did not alleviate the problem. I found, instead of pushing these images to the back of my mind, I would bravely visualise each nightmare – run through each of them in my mind before I went to sleep. I found the nightmares would not reappear. As I recall, the nightmares were not of personality conflicts or projection issues, they were more of monsters and shadowy, unrecognizable, abstract forms. I was born directly at the end of World War 2 and the dark energies this world conflict caused were deeply entrenched in my family's psyche and in the population generally, and the world around me after I was conceived and born. It could even have been energy passing from my grandfather who was in the trenches in France, in World War 1. I knew him for only the first 12 months of my life. In that same 12 months my father returned from WW2 and lost his mother as well as his father.

Do we have control over these shadows appearing? Why do we invite and promote through drama and art the very themes that conflict us? It's universal and it would seem, it appears to be essential to our inner balance

However, fear causes all types of human reactions, some find controlling others, blaming others, preaching, contrived good works, violence and racial discord a panacea or distraction. None of this is really necessary if we understand the shadows, befriend them, expose them, accept and trust their necessity, as we do in kid's stories and adult dramas. These dark shadowy episodes that persist and are invited complement the light, and make our existence whole.

Some days we wake up in a flat mood. This is sometimes referred to as 'getting out of the wrong side of bed.' Putting aside health issues, chemical influences and simply dietary indiscretions, during the night shadowy images can come forward from various levels of our unconscious, sometimes unrecognizable, affecting us for hours, days or longer. We may not even remember the dreams that affected us.

It is not unusual for us to clearly experience precognitive dreams outlining positive and negative events in the future, which our unconscious, without the tainting and restraining drawbacks (filtering) of our ego. Some may call these experiences psychic, some understand the powers of the unconscious without the restraints of the ego are limitless both in dark and light realms.

How can we turn negative energies into positive? Simply do not fear the dark. Recognise the various energies, understand them and their place in the contrasting realities of life and growth. Embrace them, vent them and realise in some cases we are not responsible for those energies passed down through time – both positive and negative.

Violence and mayhem in human adult entertainment almost seem obligatory. Even stories for the very young also have shadowy troll figures. What would a story be without the dark side? Hollywood knows all about that and how to take us to the edge and bring us back just in time, most times. Shadowy individuals on the internet are the modern mythical energies we have named trolls. They pop out from beneath the cyber bridge and do their devilish rants.

Is there a connection between the shadowy figures in children's books, adult horror movies and actual destruction? No, there is a major difference with entertainment we can experience and put back into the 'non-real' box of the past and entertainment. There are some minds that can't differentiate fiction and reality and their brain runs with the negative and the positive. It seems to be a fact that we have a need to go to those shadowy spaces as long as we can put those images away at will – switch them off. It is important to think about the age-old saying 'there is nothing to fear but fear itself.' The tricky part is signalling out shadowy energies and looking at them individually. It is in their combined state they fool and control us. (Refer Chapter 5, The Blues.)

Fears, as with many other human recollections, can be distorted and titillated. We tend to dramatise. Most recorded periods of history are of conflict. The peaceful periods of human existence, between conflicts, are less recorded and don't make the headlines. Why is this? Generally, there seems to be a human preoccupation with negative news and those prepared to exploit it.

It all starts with us as individuals. Can we watch the news objectively? Can we have peaceful periods without constant drama, be it self-created or fictionalised in film and books? Can we cross the troll's bridges without being spooked? Can we refrain unconsciously from disturbing the reactive trolls and pass quietly on our way?

Can we have compassion for the angry trolls, look them in the eye and put out a brave hand of empathic, firm understanding?

Yes, this is all possible when feelings are vented with a trusted friend, or counsellor or mentor. Eventually with patience, experience and discipline the rays of trust, empathy, compassion and acceptance will shine from the heart through the darkest of clouds.

Can we fly with the angels? At least sometimes.

CHAPTER
10

THE BIG MOVERS

We often feel we create and control most, if not all, our driving energies. Deep within us at very early ages there appears to be many specific and universal drives that appear spontaneously. These energies, which are very specific, are generally accepted as normal. From early childhood and through the rest of our lives we are moved by these powerful forces, most times without consciously knowing why.

From the time we are born we are constantly modelling behaviours around us, however children under the age of three will still surprise us with very pronounced spontaneous, specific, universal behaviours which seem beyond the child, surfacing from deep within their unconscious, gently, steadily, sometimes ruthlessly pushing and motivating them.

The drives that can appear organically and manifest in children and adults can include; need for shelter, to produce, to trade, to grow plants, to nurture, to hunt, to protest, to be territorial, instinctive sexual exploration, to compete, to love, affection and warmth, adventure and artistically create, to wonder with nature, to nourish, to strive for balance, hero worship and projection and accumulate materially.

As we develop, fear, greed, insecurities and pride can begin to distort the innocent energies and games of early childhood. They change and can become distorted or refined into something very special.

Some children get a head start as if they are directly taking off from where previous gifted individuals, both positive and negative, have left off. This phenomenon can display itself in many ways, sometimes we just nod and take it for granted.

It is difficult to distinguish between modelled behaviours and those that come from deep instinctive levels. Generally, we experience a combination of both. We can however, observe from childhood, certain energies that surface without the influence of our environment and modelling, however this can always be disputed.

The nurturing energies are very evident at a very early age. Soft toys and dolls seem to be compelling accessories for the very young. The development of the ego, even in babies, although encouraged by significant others, seems, in many cases, to be self-motivating and strong.

Sexual instincts can be present at a very early age. These energies in the very young can surprise and sometimes distress some adults with projected guilt. The need to investigate can begin at a very early age.

The instinctive drive for security and individual development demonstrates itself in the need for a hut or cubby house. Adults can be included or specifically barred from these very compelling and private games. This territorialism in later life can display itself in broader, cultural, religious disputes and war.

Creativity is another energy that wells up automatically reflecting the immediate environment, but also energies which come from much deeper areas of the psyche.

Many children's stories contain heroes and heroines which seem to be innately present. It's debatable whether movies or stories, do instigate these energies or just follow and add to pre-existing innate instinctive embedded forces. Combined with the hero energies, the need for weapons and physical assertiveness appears deep from within the psyche or a combination of innate and modelling.

To reproduce, could be argued, is passed on genetically. This very strong force appears at very early ages, seemingly too strong and premature to be a learnt behaviour.

We can go back to the child, not just as an older age retreat, but as a refreshing return to original exciting childhood instincts and magical outcomes. If you are young this may seem quite an unusual claim, but if sensitive, this may unfold as the years go by. We can choose to look forward to the regurgitation of these beautiful experiences or add them to our list of fears, for the future.

Meanwhile, the child of the universe, armed with instincts, stands at the top of the pyramid of time, relentlessly readying itself for the countless generations to come.

CHAPTER
11

CONFRONTATION WITH THE UNCONSCIOUS (UNIVERSE)

The unconscious with all its light and dark is prone to exaggeration and distortion. But, relentlessly delivers the paradoxes of life according to the background, perceptions, imagination, creativity, relative sensitivity, personal symbology of the individual and the collective unconscious.

The unconscious, at its numerous levels, all overlap and intermingle. From archetypal forces, instinctive drives, ancestral, community energies, religious influences, to personal developed cause and effect, not to completely discount the possibility of extra-terrestrial influences.

At some point in the development of an individual journey, this incredible collection of ebbing and flowing latent positive and negative energies may need to be examined and confronted. These complex, overlapping, potent life forces are a potpourri of everything within each of us. Unwrapping the unconscious could be likened to opening Pandora's Box, the abyss or, at the other extreme, transcendence to heaven. Wars, and conflicts back through time; all the atrocities against women, children, animals and men still remain powerful background energies. Although, once faced, these very atrocities crystalise into fears and shadows, and can actually compliment the seeming positives. It would seem men and women's free will remains the importance of the higher self, in spite of its perverse outcomes. If we consider all humans as brothers and sisters, it is inevitable we move past paternal empathy to actually feeling empathy. However, the responsibility for restraint and discipline is far from that of the ego, the Universe, *God or the Higher self.* Collective and individual free will, needs to, and will, run its course. This is very evident.

Unwrapping the positive and negative forces of the unconscious can be a perilous undertaking. Some recreational drug induced people visit these realms and the results can be overwhelming, if not fatal.

There are no shortcuts.

In my book Fine Line, (as referenced earlier) one protagonist, Geoffrey Blake, unwittingly takes this journey. In chapter 6 of my novel Fine Line, Blake enters a warehouse and attempts to travel the centre cobblestoned path with all the ferocities of life, symbolically to his left and right. If he moves to either extreme, he faces the attacks of negative forces symbolised by chained wild animals. With a light in the distance, he reaches a cross-road and his instinctive Neanderthal man crosses in front of him, with indifference. He later reconciles with this ancient human form. He accepts and has empathy for his inner instinctive man, which the Neanderthal represents. This being a negative experience, but with positive outcomes.

We are all visited by nightmares, dreams of projected images, scenarios, dreams of feelings, precognitive dreams and spiritual dreams. Biblical leaders use dreams. Tribal medicine and modern-day psychologists use dreams as windows into an individual's unconscious. Or, some controversial politicians use unconscious negative fears, guilts and projected prejudice to divide individuals, states and nations. Some cults tend to operate in a similar fashion.

Civil rights leader Martin Luther King said 'I had a dream; I have been to the mountaintop.' But most leaders are selective, they do not put forward their personal nightmares. However, from the top of his mountain dream, King may have experienced negatives and positives as complimentary paradoxes.

I can put forward a nightmare of my own, which I experienced in my early twenties. I was swimming in a warm pool. I had the feeling of being stalked under the water. Something grabbed my leg and pulled me under. I could see it was a dark shadow. I struggled to reach the surface, I could not. When I finally surfaced, I could see the pool attendant reading a magazine and accused him, in my mind, of not watching the safety of the pool.

In my twenties, I put this dream forward in a seminar, not really understanding it, but realised it was highly important to my development. My mentor, who was lecturing asked me 'Noel, could you breathe under the water?' I answered, 'yes'. He went on to say the dark stalker was my unconscious mythical shadow. The inattentive pool attendant represents my projected guilty ego.

In life we all add to our shadow. The degree of intent, innocence and negligent repetition adds to the size and density of our shadow. The shadow, shadows of others and shadows from past generations can combine and create an impenetrable barrier for an individual seeking truth. Fear nourishes the negative ego and enables it to flourish even against our conscious will.

We are all a product of what we create, but also what has gone before us. We sit at the top of the human pyramid. All previous experiences are focussed on us and this can be quite a burden to bear. Sometimes it is too much. We need to delineate between what we have put into motion and what was put into effect before we were born. This is practically impossible for it can be an abyss and extremely complex, further complicated by sensitivity and stage of development of each individual.

Some would say live in the now, live a life of distraction, or be part of a group for security. For others, there's no simple answer. However, paradoxically, the answers are simple and they are within each of us.

For some, a journey to the edge of the abyss is a necessary journey. To go into the abyss one can be lost forever.

Can we venture out into the solar system, or is the Milky Way the limit? Sometimes, maybe the here and now is all we have.

If we settle into the here and now without knowing how we arrived, it could be likened to an ostrich with its head in the sand. The universe is in constant flux and sand keeps moving.

We cannot trust blindly, nor can we lose ourselves in the darkness and light of the past. The paradox of darkness and light has been a driving force in our evolution, and that of the universe. Many great civilisations acknowledge the past. To evolve is to be aware of what has preceded us, dark and light, then move on. If true empathy for the contexts of the past can be generated, an individual can do no more. And yet, much more.

With brave hearts, we are born to learn how to accept.

CHAPTER
12

IN THE ARMS OF THE UNIVERSE

Life is a continual process of acceptance. We experience happiness and sorrow, pain and gratification, dark and light, prosperity and poverty, health and sickness, life and death. Just when we feel we have managed to bundle things into some semblance of order, the next moment it can all seem to crash down around us. The perceptions, the habits of our ego, the identification with our physical form, psychological make-up and our nature, can be at cross purposes with the continual process of us accepting people, our real higher selves, the world of opposites we live in and the natural catastrophes of an ever-changing dynamic earth and universe we are actually made of.

Is there any magical way we can guarantee our health, happiness, life span and relationships? No there is not. What then can we do to cope with everything in our life and previous generations, which we have no control over? Sure, following a righteous path does lessen some negative situations in life, if we don't smoke or drink alcohol, eat the right foods, forgive and care about others and avoid taking risks, we moderate certain consequences. But, even if we attempt to do everything 'right' and tell the truth to the best of our ability, we are not immune, especially from the natural and human accelerated catastrophes of the environment we exist in. The process of the complimenting opposites will test our perceptions, our personal, physical and universal spirit.

How do we know what we can and cannot change?

Our personal existence, many times, seems to be diametrically opposed to the way of nature and the universe. To accept the difference and paradoxes of the 'positive' and 'negative' forces in this world, may be one of our finest endeavours.

The higher self within each of us, seems to hold all the cards. We are in its hands and arms of the universal spirit whether we want to admit it or not. If we are patient and trust, in time, amazing things can happen, although not necessarily in our relatively short lifetimes. If we resist the laws of the universe at the individual level or at the cultural level, the conflict within and projected outward will be strikingly obvious, if not to us, to others consciously and unconsciously. This is not the universe or God's doing – it is ours, although we should not be too tough on ourselves. We are developing individuals and we all have free will, which involves mistakes and pain. When I was younger, I referred to my own stubbornness in this way, 'The thicker the skull, the bigger the brick.'

On the slopes of the unpredictable volcano Mt Vesuvius, Naples, below the constant smoking summit, farmers live on and cultivate the rich, fertile volcanic soils, accepting the periodical eruptions of the volcano. The souvenir stores, and the kiosks situated at the ever-smoking summit, which I have visited, are all fitted with wheels so they can be towed away quickly if an eruption is imminent.

The serene surface of our dark and light planet, can, if we let it, lull us into a false sense of security. Just forty to sixty kilometres below the surface, a molten fury exists and on a continual basis, in various parts of the world, the fiery centre of the earth comes to the surface and the fury of the ever-changing universe can manifest itself right on our doorstep. We sometimes build huge cities along these volcanic fault lines. Deep within our psyche we accept the possible consequences, however, when eruptions occur, those affected are usually devastated.

Sometimes out of nowhere some nasty thoughts can erupt the surface of our minds. Very potent, these thoughts, sometimes in the form of way-out dreams, which are out of character with our normal thinking, could come from ancestry influences or possibly what is referred to as the deeper, collective, instinctive human psyche. All thoughts that enter our minds are electrical impulses and do not amount to anything unless we act on them. Extremes of the mind both aspirational and devilish can be observed, accepted and this process of balance can add to our inner growth.

Constantly, the human psyche with the negative guidance of leaders who use division, cultural disharmony and prejudice, selfishness and fear, stir the fiery ego core of the human condition, setting men and women against each other, causing division, wars and suffering. However, time and time again it has been proven people can be fooled some of the time, but not all of the people all of the time.

In a lecture I once attended, the crucifixion of Christ was put forward as an example of the conflict between the 'higher self' and the human ego. 'The vertical upright of the cross represented 'God's way', the way of the universe. The horizontal, was likened to men and women's way – the way of the human ego. Jesus was nailed where the vertical and horizontal timbers crossed.'

To have an ego is very human and a privilege, however we only have to look at our own lives and the various influential individual egos of the world, past and present, to understand the negative and sometimes evil energies that these individuals can generate. It continues to this very day. We all contribute daily, in some way, to the world ego. Do we add to the energies of greed, division and prejudice, or do we promote balance and harmony (honest, caring, a relaxed and nonjudgmental existence)? We probably have to accept that we are materialistically minded, because we may well be. Balance within a relative environment, using innate abilities to prosper, and to consider others at the same time, is possible.

It has been said the positive or negative condition of one leaf on a tree, in some way, affects the whole tree.

Many of the great sages and religions of the world speak of the pitfalls of material, physical and psychological attachment. We have all experienced the loss of something or somebody we love. The pain can be excruciating. To love deeply and remain detached is probably one of the most difficult of human experiences. It is understandable why so many of us are apprehensive to show our feelings, and just sit on the fence.

It is so amazing how things are taken for granted and it does not take very long at all, after reaching a feeling of 'happiness,' to rush on seeking more and more. Is this wrong? No, it's a normal human reaction. We progress as civilizations and individuals in this way. Many on this planet do not have the luxury of feeling 'happy' and cannot move onto bigger and better lives. But even in some of the humblest human conditions people do find contentment.

Coming to terms with reality is not the same for a Brit as it is for an African. It is not the same for the Russians as for an Inuit. It would not be the same for a Neanderthal as for an American living in contemporary America. For intelligent life that may exist on other planets, acceptance of their lives and ways may be far different from that of humans.

Acceptance of our material lot in life can be a relative state of mind. It can be found in the humblest of human conditions and, although more challenging, it can manifest itself in affluent societies. Common to all socio-economic groups, acceptance of death, loss of physical and mental health, is an equal challenge to every individual person on the planet. The number of possessions, or position in society, as we know, gives no sanctions.

Acceptance can be coloured and influenced by religion, by race, by culture, gender, age, sexual orientation, sickness and physical challenges. It is a dynamic, daily, changing reality. Within the individual the process of acceptance changes daily in positive and negative trends. In the wider community and at the cultural levels, evolved acceptance, through religion and education and collective experience, guides most of the population. The opposing laws of the universe (or God) continually tests any ego that exists within it. Acceptance can be intellectualised, idealised, it can be preached, or it can be a natural growing life friend.

A person who is imprisoned for life, told they have only months to live, or somebody facing immediate execution, all face varying time frames of reality. Acceptance is a continually, non-static, changing phenomena. Sometimes we can understand and accept, sometimes we can dogmatically find peace and sometimes we will be swept away by circumstances and hold on tightly as the roller coaster of life goes through its cycles.

There are times, regardless of whatever preparation we go through – we can lose control. Ultimately trust is all we can experience. Trust in the essence and continuation of life, the innate goodness that is evident throughout all cultures and the seeming contradictory patterns of the universe/God.

Carl Jung wrote 'when one follows the path of individualization (a path seeking personal truth). As one lives his or her life, one must take mistakes into the bargain. Life would not be complete without them. There is no guarantee, not for one moment we will not fall into fatal error or stumble into deadly peril. We may think there is a sure road, but that may be the downward road.' (Jung, 1963)

Once we accept and trust, things can open up. Once we hit what seems to be the bottom, that can in fact be the positive pinnacle in reverse. After attempting to bend life to suit our perceptions, which have been fashioned in our lifetime and passed on from previous generations, other parallel generations and cultural influences, we find reality, the universe, and God allows us to run with free will until we can go no further. When we either are stubborn or trust within the bounds of our well-meaning perceptions, want an answer, answers will come when we are ready. How we react and perform up to the point of being given these gifts decides the amount of physical and mental pain we will experience. In other words, we can go easy to truth or we can resist and experience varying health and mental traumas. These seeming consequences can be blessings in disguise.

The contemporary musical Jesus Christ Superstar demonstrates a fascinating perception of the writers. In one particular scene where Jesus is on the cross, he cries out, 'Do what you want with me Lord, you hold all the cards.' Jesus could be saying, according to the writers, 'I understand my perceptions are limited.'

We exist in our conscious and unconscious world. We see what goes on in our daily conscious world, but only through intuition, dreams, meditation, prayer and the arts do we get a glimpse at the unconscious world with its complimenting dark and light sides. Acceptance that there are things we cannot grasp and understand is vital. This is where trust comes in, trust that a universal spirit of goodwill, goodwill based on, and displayed through how we rear our young, will transcend negative forces and those that have the sad ability to see the dark side of the unconscious and use it for their own selfish means. We only have to travel this world we live in to experience, at the grassroots level, the raw goodness, friendship and reflective love we receive and give to all cultures we visit.

We are in the arms of the universe, but a universe which does not centre around us. We are all made up of pieces of the universe. Time is of the universe, not our perceived reality. Our personal time density is directly relative to the understanding of how our ego limits us. We only have to look up at the night sky to see, feel and experience our origin. If we look inward, a microcosm of the universe will be evident to each of us. Only clouds in the sky and clouds in our minds hold us back temporarily from constant viewing higher realities and occurrences.

As with humans, animals, plants and all that be, the magical other side underpins all things and directly influences behaviours and physical existence. As we attempt to follow a path of truth, the universal and godly energies are constantly running in parallel, blending, complementing, challenging and are completely unpredictable.

Even truth can be paradoxically tested by natural organic realities.

When all is done, even at the highest level of human perceptual interpretations, realities such as human conflict, cyclones, earthquakes, natural human ageing and death, are common denominators of our existence.

I spoke to my dog, lying beside me whilst I was writing.

'Little Masie, you don't seem to be influenced by these paradoxes, you live in the here and now.' She looked at me as if to say 'I know, but I have my limits – you have much more – use it wisely and don't get too distracted.'

'Let's play ball.'

Acknowledgements

Thank you to my many mentors who all appeared at the times I needed them in my life.

Thank you to those individuals who have challenged me, usually with aspects of themselves not unlike some of my own.

Thank you to Bella Macdonald for her support.

Thank you to Emma my editor.

Thank you to Blaise and Kev at Busybird Publishing.

References

Jung, Carl. *Memories, Dreams and Reflections.* Vintage Books, Random House, 1963

Doidge, Norman. *The Brain's Way of Healing.* Scribe, 2015

Walker, Matthew. *Why We Sleep.* Random House, 2017

Willis, Lilly. '*The Psychic Side of Churchill.*' Psychics Directory, https://www.psychicsdirectory.com/articles/winston-churchill_and_psychics/

www.ingramcontent.com/pod-product-compliance
Lightning Source LLC
Chambersburg PA
CBHW071738080526
44588CB00013B/2075